T0189460

Cancer Drug Discovery and Development

Series Editor
Beverly A. Teicher
Bethesda, Maryland, USA

More information about this series at http://www.springer.com/series/7625

Massimo Cristofanilli

Editor

Liquid Biopsies in Solid Tumors

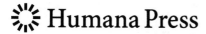 Humana Press

Editor
Massimo Cristofanilli
Department of Medicine-Hematology and Oncology
Robert H. Lurie Comprehensive Cancer Center
Northwestern University
Chicago, IL, USA

ISSN 2196-9906   ISSN 2196-9914   (electronic)
Cancer Drug Discovery and Development
ISBN 978-3-319-84530-2   ISBN 978-3-319-50956-3   (eBook)
DOI 10.1007/978-3-319-50956-3

Printed on acid-free paper

This Humana Press imprint is published by Springer Nature
The registered company is Springer International Publishing AG
The registered company address is: Gewerbestrasse 11, 6330 Cham, Switzerland

Preface

Solid tumors have been traditionally evaluated using a combination of anatomic, pathological, and radiological tools. The AJCC staging classification provides important prognostic information for planning treatment modalities. In reality, cancer is a disease characterized by complex genomic changes (e.g., mutations, gene rearrangements) resulting in activating pathways associated with treatment resistance and disease progression. Furthermore, an additional level of complexity is represented by tumor heterogeneity, particularly in the metastatic setting due to the existence of cancer cell clones with distinct biological features. Molecular diagnostics has evolved allowing the *real-time* assessment of cancer complexity by a simple blood test to interrogate the "liquid phase" of solid tumors. A revolutionary approach to cancer diagnostics that complements and expands the role of standard pathology. Today, liquid biopsy technologies allow to collect circulating cancer cells or DNA fragments representative of the disease but also expression of resistance clones seeding various metastatic sites providing clinicians with the advantage to understand, predict, and intervene. In this book, we have collected contribution from experts in the field of blood-based diagnostics to present the silent diagnostic revolution and the perspectives and impact on patients' management. The future of cancer early detection, characterization, and monitoring using liquid biopsies will mirror the management of chronic diseases such as diabetes and hypercholesterolemia.

Chicago, IL, USA

Massimo Cristofanilli

Contents

1 **Blood-Based Diagnostics in Solid Tumors: An Overview** 1
   Angela Toss and Massimo Cristofanilli

2 **Circulating Tumour Cells in Primary Disease:**
   The Seed for Metastasis 15
   Noam Falbel Pondé and Michail Ignatiadis

3 **Enumeration and Molecular Analysis of CTCs**
   in Metastatic Disease: The Breast Cancer Model 41
   Cleo Parisi and Evi Lianidou

4 **Epithelial-Mesenchymal Transition (EMT) and Cancer Stem**
   Cells (CSCs): The Traveling Metastasis 67
   Michal Mego, James Reuben, and Sendurai A. Mani

5 **Detecting and Monitoring Circulating Stromal Cells**
   from Solid Tumors Using Blood-Based Biopsies
   in the Twenty-First Century: Have Circulating Stromal Cells
   Come of Age? 81
   Daniel L. Adams and Massimo Cristofanilli

6 **Circulating Free Tumor DNA (ctDNA): The Real-Time**
   Liquid Biopsy 105
   Kelly Kyker-Snowman and Ben Ho Park

7 **CTCs and ctDNA: Two Tales of a Complex Biology** 119
   Paul W. Dempsey

8 **Exosomes: The Next Small Thing** 139
   Vincent J. O'Neill

Index 157

Contributors

Daniel L. Adams Creatv MicroTech, Inc., Monmouth Junction, NJ, USA

Massimo Cristofanilli Robert H. Lurie Comprehensive Cancer Center, Northwestern University, Chicago, IL, USA

Paul W. Dempsey, Ph.D. Cynvenio Biosystems Inc., Westlake Village, CA, USA

Michail Ignatiadis Department of Medical Oncology, Institut Jules Bordet, Boulevard de Waterloo, Brussels, Belgium

Kelly Kyker-Snowman The Sidney Kimmel Comprehensive Cancer Center, The Johns Hopkins University School of Medicine, Baltimore, MD, USA

Evi Lianidou Department of Chemistry, Laboratory of Analytical Chemistry, Analysis of Circulating Tumor Cells (ACTC) Lab, University of Athens, Athens, Greece

Sendurai A. Mani Department of Translational Molecular Pathology, Division of Pathology/Lab Medicine, The University of Texas MD Anderson Cancer Center, Houston, TX, USA

Michal Mego National Cancer Institute, Bratislava, Slovak Republic

Department of Oncology, Faculty of Medicine, Comenius University and National Cancer Institute, Bratislava, Slovakia

Vincent J. O'Neill, M.D. Mirna Therapeutics, Austin, TX, USA

Cleo Parisi Department of Chemistry, Laboratory of Analytical Chemistry, Analysis of Circulating Tumor Cells (ACTC) Lab, University of Athens, Athens, Greece

Ben Ho Park The Sidney Kimmel Comprehensive Cancer Center, The Johns Hopkins University School of Medicine, Baltimore, MD, USA

Department of Chemical and Biomolecular Engineering, The Johns Hopkins University, Baltimore, MD, USA

Noam Falbel Pondé Department of Medical Oncology, Institut Jules Bordet, Boulevard de Waterloo, Brussels, Belgium

James Reuben Department of Hematopathology, Division of Pathology/Lab Medicine, The University of Texas MD Anderson Cancer Center, Houston, TX, USA

Angela Toss Department of Oncology and Haematology, University of Modena and Reggio Emilia, Modena, Italy

Chapter 1
Blood-Based Diagnostics in Solid Tumors: An Overview

Angela Toss and Massimo Cristofanilli

Abstract The application of patient-specific genetic information and molecular tumor characteristics enables the selection of treatment strategies for individual patients, improving the therapeutic efficacy and expanding the scope of personalized medicine. Emerging evidence from clinical research provides demonstration that the genetic landscape of any given tumor will dictate its sensitivity or resistance profile to anticancer agents. Nevertheless, the inter- and intra-tumor genetic heterogeneity can be a substantial impediment to the successful clinical application of this approach. Since acquired drug resistance is common during the course of the disease, there is an urgent need to monitor tumor evolution. On these bases, the importance of molecular re-characterization of metastatic disease has been prospectively confirmed and has been recently acknowledged in the clinical guidelines for the management of advanced malignancies. Nevertheless, obtaining serial samples of metastatic tissue is impractical and complicated by spatial heterogeneity, sampling bias, and invasive procedures. An attractive alternative to overcome these limitations is represented by the analysis of peripheral blood sample as a "liquid biopsy." Blood draws can easily be performed serially; thus blood would be an ideal compartment for detection of prognostic and predictive biomarkers. Nowadays, the principal sources for liquid biopsies are represented by cells and intracellular materials that are released by the tumor mass and are swept away by the bloodstream, such as CTCs, ctDNA, and exosomes. This book provides an overview of the technological approaches to perform and enhance the strategy and the principal applications in clinical practice of "liquid biopsy."

Keywords Tumor heterogeneity • Liquid biopsy • Circulating tumor cell • Circulating tumor DNA • Exosome

A. Toss
Department of Oncology and Haematology, University of Modena and Reggio Emilia, Modena 41121, Italy

M. Cristofanilli (✉)
Robert H. Lurie Comprehensive Cancer Center, Northwestern University, Chicago, IL 60611, USA
e-mail: Massimo.Cristofanilli@nm.org

© Springer International Publishing AG 2017   1
M. Cristofanilli (ed.), *Liquid Biopsies in Solid Tumors*, Cancer Drug Discovery and Development, DOI 10.1007/978-3-319-50956-3_1

The standard of care for many patients with advanced solid tumors is gradually evolving from the empirical selection of treatments to the use of targeted approaches based on the immunohistochemical and molecular profile of the tumor. In the last decade, an increasing number of therapeutic agents targeting molecular abnormalities have been developed for the treatment of solid tumors [1]. Several of them have been already approved for the use in daily clinical practice (i.e., trastuzumab, everolimus, gefitinib, pazopanib) while many still remain in the context of clinical trials (i.e., BKM120, BYL719) [2]. These drugs target specific genomic abnormalities associated with gain of function or downstream signal activation including mutated protein kinases and amplified or rearranged transcription factors. These alterations, called "*driver mutations*," confer to cancer cells a survival advantage and thus targeting these alterations is a rational strategy to offer more personalized and effective treatment to metastatic patients. Particularly, the term "*personalized medicine*" refers to the application of patient-specific genetic information and molecular and/ or cellular tumor characteristics to select the optimal treatment for individual patients with the goal of improved therapeutic efficacy. Therefore, the identification of predictive biomarkers is important both to spare nonresponders from the side effects associated with treatment and to minimize the overall cost by increasing therapeutic ratio for patients with advanced malignancies.

Emerging evidence from clinical trials assessing targeted therapies provides demonstration that the genetic landscape of any given tumor will dictate its sensitivity or resistance profile to anticancer agents [3]. Nevertheless, the inter- and intratumor genetic heterogeneity can be a substantial impediment to the successful clinical application of this approach. Previous studies demonstrated that cancer is a dynamic and heterogeneous entity following the principles of clonal evolution, with different areas of the same primary tumor showing different genomic profiles and with metastases acquiring new molecular aberrations as compared to their primary tumors [4–7].

Different models have been proposed to explain the origins of this heterogeneity (Fig. 1.1) [8–10]:

1. The "clonal evolution theory", proposed by Nowell in 1976, suggests that tumor masses are caused by the expansion of one (monoclonal) or multiple (polyclonal) cellular subpopulations of clones. In this egalitarian model, heritable changes in the epigenome can confer advantageous traits on variant subpopulations, allowing their clonal expansion. In this model, the selection pressures imposed by the tumor microenvironment can selectively favor clones with more malignant phenotypes (according to the Darwinian model) [11].
2. In the "mutator hypothesis," tumor mass develops because of the gradual and random accumulation of genetic mutations, causing a wide range of diversity [12].
3. In the "cancer stem cell (CSC) model," some precursor cells give rise to a different subpopulation of cells within the tumor with a hierarchical arrangement. According to this model, CSCs reside at the apex of a cellular hierarchy and are capable of undergoing self-renewal to generate daughters that once again exhibit

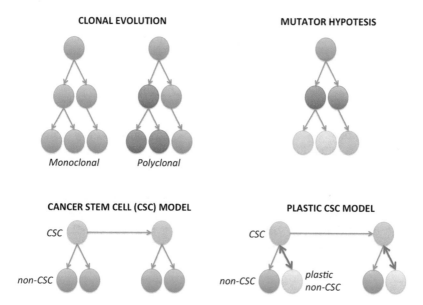

Fig. 1.1 Different models at the basis of tumor heterogeneity

the CSC phenotype. Alternatively, they can undergo asymmetric division to create daughters (non-CSCs) with limited tumorigenic and metastatic potential that have initiated differentiation programs. A central concept of the CSC model is that a small subpopulation of cells within a tumor drives the growth and progression of the tumor as a whole, while, in established tumors, the non-CSCs, being in the great majority, are responsible for expressing many of the phenotypic traits that determine the traits of the tumor as a whole [13–15].

4. In the last few years, a plastic "cancer stem cell model" has been developed. According to this alternative hypothesis, committed non-CSCs can undergo a dedifferentiation process and reenter the CSC state with the capacity for self-renewal and the ability to efficiently reconstitute differentiated tumors. Therefore, the emerging model suggests that tumors can originate from the transformation of normal adult tissue stem cells or from more differentiated progenitors that have acquired stem-like capabilities [15, 16].

The clonal heterogeneity, exacerbated by the selective pressures imposed by treatment during the life cycle of the disease, is able to confer greater resistance to anticancer treatments and radiation therapy [17]. Multiple lines of evidence showed relevant rates of discordance between the phenotype of primary tumor and that of subsequent metastatic disease, confirming the concept of intra-tumor heterogeneity [18–20]. Since acquired drug resistance is common during the course of the disease, there is an urgent need to monitor tumor evolution and ideally predict the onset of resistance to targeted therapies. On these bases, the importance of molecular re-characterization of metastatic disease has been prospectively confirmed [21] and it has been recently acknowledged in the clinical guidelines for the management of advanced malignancies. Since therapy-related biomarkers may change throughout tumor progression "in time and space," the measurement of the biomarker of interest at multiple time points and different sites of metastasis may provide crucial information for patient management. However, in routine clinical practice the re-characterization of metastases for the evaluation of biomarkers predicting therapy response is nowadays provided by invasive tumor biopsies. Therefore, obtaining serial samples of metastatic tissue is impractical and complicated by spatial heterogeneity and sampling bias. More comprehensive and accessible tumor genome information is needed to provide an accurate portrait of the whole tumor than those that can be offered by a single biopsy. An attractive alternative to overcome the limitation of repeated tissue sampling is represented by the analysis of peripheral blood sample as a "*liquid biopsy*." Cancer patients undergoing treatment frequently undergo blood draws for various diagnostic and treatment-monitoring reasons. Blood draws can easily be performed serially; thus blood would be an ideal compartment for detection of metastatic tumor cells.

Circulating Biomarkers in the Peripheral Blood

A typical primary tumor contains millions or even billions of cells harboring genetic mutations that drive them to grow, divide, and invade the surrounding tissues. Some of these cells slough off the edges of the tumor mass and are swept away by the bloodstream or lymphatic system. These cells can remain loose in circulation, cluster together as they travel, or lodge themselves in new tissues, creating distant metastases [22]. One of the most important determinants of prognosis and management of cancer patients is the absence or presence of this metastatic dissemination at the time of initial presentation or during treatments [23, 24]. The spread of tumor cells to lymph nodes or bone marrow is referred to as "disseminated tumor cells (DTCs)," and as "circulating tumor cells (CTCs)" when present in the peripheral blood [25].

In the last decade, the detection of CTCs in the blood has demonstrated to provide useful information for the clinical management of metastatic solid tumors. Moreover, other potential blood-based markers are emerging as independent parameters for prediction of development and outcome in metastatic disease, including circulating tumor microemboli and circulating tumor materials (CTMat). The apoptosis and necrosis processes of CTCs cause the leakage of intracellular components in the bloodstream, such as electrolytes, cellular debris, DNA, and chromatin. Since CTCs are continuously released and destroyed, such CTMat accumulate and could represent an independent biomarker for the prognostication and monitoring of metastatic disease.

Nowadays, the principal sources for liquid biopsies are represented by CTCs, ctDNA, and exosomes.

Circulating Tumor Cells (CTCs)

The presence of tumor cells in the peripheral circulation of a man with metastatic cancer was reported for the first time in 1869 by Thomas Ashworth [26]. In 1955, Engell observed a larger frequency of tumor cells in the draining vein of the tumor as compared to the peripheral blood [27]. In the late 1970s, the introduction of sensitive and specific immunohistochemical techniques renewed the interest in the CTC detection and their possible association with early metastasization in solid malignancies [28]. Since then, proofs of CTCs in the blood from patients with metastatic and primary carcinoma were found by immunohistochemistry staining. In the 1990s, CTCs were found in neuroblastoma patients and in patients with colorectal, breast, small-cell, and non-small-cell lung cancer [29–31]. These studies demonstrated that tumor cells can be detected by traditional immunochemistry techniques but also that traditional immunochemistry lacks the sensitivity to be used in larger multicenter studies.

Tumor cells in blood are present in a high background of hematopoietic cells and are found at a very low concentration even in patients with metastatic disease [32]. Moreover, one of the problems in the development of assays to detect these rare cells is not knowing whether tumor cells are present, and if so at what frequency. Therefore, CTC detection and characterization require highly sensitive and specific methods, which consist of a combination of enrichment (isolation) and detection (identification) strategies and both steps are essential components of the identification process [33]. Enrichment techniques are based on two different strategies: the selection according to morphological features (size, density, electric charges, deformability) or according to immunologic profile (cell surface protein expression such as EpCAM). After enrichment, the solution usually still contains several leukocytes; thus CTCs need to be identified at the single-cell level and separated from normal blood cells. CTC detection can be done through cytometric strategies (immunocytochemistry) or nucleic acid-based techniques (PCR, RT-PCR) [1]. However, for any technology to be used in the clinic, demonstration of analytic validity (the accuracy of the test to measure the target of interest), clinical validity (the value of the test to predict the clinical outcome), and ultimately clinical utility (ability of the test to lead to improved clinical outcome when treatment choice is informed by test results) is required [34–36]. The only system currently approved by the FDA in monitoring patients with metastatic breast, colorectal, or prostate cancer is CellSearch (Janssen Diagnostics) [37, 38]. The first clinical studies conducted with the CellSearch system showed that CTCs are clearly associated with poor prognosis in metastatic breast, colorectal, and castration-resistant prostate cancer. Moreover, later studies showed the same for small-cell lung cancer and non-small-cell lung cancer (NSCLC), bladder cancer, pancreas cancer, head and neck cancer, ovarian cancer, neuroendocrine cancer, and hepatocellular cancer [39, 40]. CellSearch proved to be able to detect CTCs before and after surgery for nonmetastatic breast, colorectal cancer, esophagus cancer, and bladder cancer [39, 40].

At present, the role of CTC can be mainly limited to prognostic purposes, but there is an increasing interest in the development of new techniques for their molecular characterization in order to guide treatment selection. Several studies analyzed the molecular aberrations carried by CTCs and compared their profile to that of primary tumor, trying to correlate some characteristics to disease aggressiveness and treatment response. In breast cancer, HER2 status on CTCs has been assessed with demonstration that some women with HER2-negative breast cancer may have detectable HER2-positive CTCs [41, 42]. Nevertheless, in two different studies lapatinib failed to provide objective responses in patients with metastatic breast cancer with HER2-negative primary tumors and HER2-positive or EGFR-positive CTCs [43, 44]. The ongoing phase III DETECT-III and CirCe T-DM1 trials will try to clarify the potential role of HER2-targeted therapies in this setting of patients. On the other hand, CTC protein expression has been analyzed in other tumor types. In patients with metastatic colorectal cancer, thymidylate synthase expression in CTCs has been studied as a potential marker of resistance to 5-fluorouracil [45], while androgen receptor (AR) signaling in CTCs from patients with metastatic prostate cancer has been evaluated to tailor hormonal treatment approaches [46].

Several proof-of-concept studies have demonstrated the feasibility of detecting somatic mutations in CTCs from patients with various tumor types [47–49]. For instance, in metastatic breast cancer, Fernandez et al. showed the feasibility of using CTCs for *TP53* mutation detection as a noninvasive method. In particular, CTCs from two triple-negative breast cancer patients were enriched using CellSearch system and single cell selected by DEPArray. Distinct CTC populations were found, some of which harboring the same *TP53* mutation (R110 delG), while some other showed either a different *TP53* mutation (*TP53* R110 delC) or the wild-type allele. These results indicate that CTCs could represent a noninvasive source of cancer cells for the determination of disease progression and the identification of new potential therapeutic targets [50]. Nevertheless, it remains unclear how many CTCs need to be analyzed to capture tumor heterogeneity sufficiently to predict treatment efficacy.

More recently, several groups have reported on the prognostic value of CTC clusters, called circulating tumor microemboli (CTM). Clusters captured using the CellSearch platform have been identified in more than 30% of patients with small-cell lung cancer, metastatic melanoma, breast cancer, and prostate cancer, and appear to lack apoptotic or proliferating cells, perhaps offering a survival advantage [51]. Similar to single migratory mesenchymal-like CTCs, CTC clusters appear to be enriched for mesenchymal markers [52] and may arise from oligoclonal tumor cell groups with high metastatic potential [52, 53].

Circulating tumor cells have now been proposed as surrogate biomarkers in over 270 clinical trials [54]. However, to date, CTCs have not been incorporated into routine clinical practice for management of patients with cancer. Further interventional controlled phase III trials are needed to investigate and define the role of CTC evaluation in the improvement of patient outcome and in the reduction of medical costs [55]. The future implementation of molecular and genomic characterization of CTCs as liquid biopsies will likely contribute to improve the treatment selection and thus to move toward precision medicine.

Circulating Tumor DNA (ctDNA)

The presence of circulating cell-free DNA (cfDNA) in the blood of healthy individuals was firstly reported by Mandel and Metais in 1948 [56]. There are few data available on the origin, mechanism, and rate of release of cfDNA release in the circulation. On the one hand, cfDNA is thought to originate from apoptotic and necrotic cells [57], and on the other hand, it has been suggested that all living cells actively release DNA into the circulation [58]. Interestingly, some reports indicated that the high proliferation of tumors leads to a higher degree of necrosis, corresponding to an increased release of tumor-related cfDNA, named circulating tumor DNA (ctDNA). As the tumor increases in volume, so too does the cellular turnover and hence the number of apoptotic and necrotic cells, leading to the accumulation of cellular debris and its inevitable release into the circulation [57, 59]. Discriminating ctDNA from normal cfDNA is possible since tumor DNA is characterized by the presence of mutations. These somatic mutations are present only in the genomes of cancer cells or precancerous cells and are not present in the DNA of normal healthy cells [60].

The study of ctDNA in cancer patients has several potential clinical applications:

1. *Monitoring tumor burden.* Rapid increases in ctDNA levels correspond to disease progression, while successful treatment with pharmacologic therapy or resective surgery brings to declines in levels of ctDNA [60–63]. Consequently, ctDNA level may be used as biomarker for monitoring tumor response to therapy, potentially defining ambiguous clinical scenarios like stable disease or mixed responses, and predicting treatment response early in the course of therapy.
2. *Detection of minimal residual disease.* Circulating tumor DNA is a potential biomarker of residual disease after resection or therapy with curative intent and may determine which patients will experience recurrence. Evaluation of ctDNA after surgery (6–8 weeks after surgery) may help therapeutic decision making regarding adjuvant treatments [60].
3. *Monitoring tumor heterogeneity and the emergence of molecular resistance.* ctDNA fragments are released from different parts of the tumor; thus they contain the same genetic abnormalities as those present in the primary tumor [64]. This means that ctDNA analysis may be a potential alternative to conventional tissue biopsies, and it can be used where tissue biopsies fail or cannot be performed. Particularly, ctDNA analysis may provide an overview of all the cancer cells DNA in a tumor simultaneously; therefore, this approach may be used to overcome the challenges posed by intra-tumor genetic heterogeneity and to offer noninvasive profiling for the presence of actionable mutations [65]. This molecular picture includes the dynamic changes that occur during therapy as well as the heterogeneity that emerges as a result of therapeutic selective pressure. Therefore, this information can be used to plan treatment strategies, selecting targeted therapies based on the molecular profile of the tumor or adopting alternate therapies before clinical resistance is detected.

4. *Early diagnosis of tumors.* Novel genomic methodologies for ctDNA detection, based on digital PCR and next-generation sequencing (NGS), are becoming very specific and sensitive, opening up the possibility of using ctDNA for screening in the future [66, 67]. Nevertheless, more work needs to be done in order to validate these new assays for the early detection of cancer.

Several studies have already demonstrated high concordance for selected actionable mutations between paired tumor biopsies and plasma specimens, particularly for metastatic breast, colorectal, and non-small-cell lung cancer [63, 68–73], confirming the validity of liquid biopsy as alternative to tissue biopsies in this subset of patients.

Exosomes

Exosomes are vesicles actively released by all cells, which carry RNA, DNA, and proteins and function as intercellular messengers [74–79]. Exosomes are extremely abundant in all biological fluids and can be isolated from serum, plasma, saliva, urine, and cerebrospinal fluid [80, 81]. Interestingly, exosomes demonstrated to play a role in micro-metastasization, angiogenesis, and immune modulation [82–84] and they are particularly interesting as cancer biomarkers since they are stable carriers of genetic material and proteins from their cell of origin.

This book provides an insight into the clinical significance of "liquid biopsy," and technological approaches to perform and enhance the strategy. Further, it offers an overview of the principal applications in clinical practice, and explores avenues for further research to solve unmet clinical needs.

References

1. Toss A, Cristofanilli M (2015) Molecular characterization and targeted therapeutic approaches in breast cancer. Breast Cancer Res 17:60
2. https://clinicaltrials.gov
3. Tsimberidou AM, Iskander NG, Hong DS, Wheler JJ, Falchook GS, Fu S, Piha-Paul S, Naing A, Janku F, Luthra R, Ye Y, Wen S, Berry D, Kurzrock R (2012) Personalized medicine in a phase I clinical trials program: the MD Anderson Cancer Center initiative. Clin Cancer Res 18(22):6373–6383
4. Ding L, Ellis MJ, Li S, Larson DE, Chen K, Wallis JW, Harris CC, McLellan MD, Fulton RS, Fulton LL, Abbott RM, Hoog J, Dooling DJ et al (2010) Genome remodelling in a basal-like breast cancer metastasis and xenograft. Nature 464(7291):999–1005
5. Navin N, Kendall J, Troge J, Andrews P, Rodgers L, McIndoo J, Cook K, Stepansky A, Levy D, Esposito D, Muthuswamy L, Krasnitz A, McCombie WR, Hicks J, Wigler M (2011) Tumour evolution inferred by single-cell sequencing. Nature 472(7341):90–94
6. Gerlinger M, Rowan AJ, Horswell S, Larkin J, Endesfelder D, Gronroos E, Martinez P, Matthews N, Stewart A, Tarpey P, Varela I, Phillimore B, Begum S et al (2012) Intratumor heterogeneity and branched evolution revealed by multiregion sequencing. N Engl J Med 366(10):883–892

7. Swanton C (2012) Intratumor heterogeneity: evolution through space and time. Cancer Res 72(19):4875–4882
8. Marusyk A, Polyak K (2010) Tumor heterogeneity: causes and consequences. Biochim Biophys Acta 1805(1):105–117
9. Navin NE, Hicks J (2010) Tracing the tumor lineage. Mol Oncol 4(3):267–283
10. Russnes HG, Navin N, Hicks J, Borresen-Dale AL (2011) Insight into the heterogeneity of breast cancer through next-generation sequencing. J Clin Invest 121(10):3810–3818
11. Nowell PC (1976) The clonal evolution of tumor cell populations. Science 194(4260):23–28
12. Loeb LA, Springgate CF, Battula N (1974) Errors in DNA replication as a basis of malignant changes. Cancer Res 34(9):2311–2321
13. Bonnet D, Dick JE (1997) Human acute myeloid leukemia is organized as a hierarchy that originates from a primitive hematopoietic cell. Nat Med 3(7):730–737
14. Lapidot T, Sirard C, Vormoor J, Murdoch B, Hoang T, Caceres-Cortes J, Minden M, Paterson B, Caligiuri MA, Dick JE (1994) A cell initiating human acute myeloid leukaemia after transplantation into SCID mice. Nature 367(6464):645–648
15. Marjanovic ND, Weinberg RA, Chaffer CL (2013) Cell plasticity and heterogeneity in cancer. Clin Chem 59(1):168–179
16. Mani SA, Guo W, Liao MJ, Eaton EN, Ayyanan A, Zhou AY, Brooks M, Reinhard F, Zhang CC, Shipitsin M, Campbell LL, Polyak K, Brisken C et al (2008) The epithelial-mesenchymal transition generates cells with properties of stem cells. Cell 133(4):704–715
17. Badve S, Nakshatri H (2012) Breast-cancer stem cells-beyond semantics. Lancet Oncol 13(1):e43–e48
18. Amir E, Clemons M, Purdie CA, Miller N, Quinlan P, Geddie W, Coleman RE, Freedman OC, Jordan LB, Thompson AM (2012) Tissue confirmation of disease recurrence in breast cancer patients: pooled analysis of multi-centre, multi-disciplinary prospective studies. Cancer Treat Rev 38(6):708–714
19. Liedtke C, Broglio K, Moulder S, Hsu L, Kau SW, Symmans WF, Albarracin C, Meric-Bernstam F, Woodward W, Theriault RL, Kiesel L, Hortobagyi GN, Pusztai L et al (2009) Prognostic impact of discordance between triple-receptor measurements in primary and recurrent breast cancer. Ann Oncol 20(12):1953–1958
20. Lindström LS, Karlsson E, Wilking UM, Johansson U, Hartman J, Lidbrink EK, Hatschek T, Skoog L, Bergh J (2012) Clinically used breast cancer markers such as estrogen receptor, progesterone receptor, and human epidermal growth factor receptor 2 are unstable throughout tumor progression. J Clin Oncol 30(21):2601–2608
21. de Dueñas EM, Hernández AL, Zotano AG, Carrión RM, López-Muñiz JI, Novoa SA, Rodríguez AL, Fidalgo JA, Lozano JF, Gasión OB, Carrascal EC, Capilla AH, López-Barajas IB et al (2014) Prospective evaluation of the conversion rate in the receptor status between primary breast cancer and metastasis: results from the GEICAM 2009-03 ConvertHER study. Breast Cancer Res Treat 143(3):507–515
22. Williams SC (2013) Circulating tumor cells. Proc Natl Acad Sci U S A 110(13):4861
23. Lugo TG, Braun S, Cote RJ, Pantel K, Rusch V (2003) Detection and measurement of occult disease for the prognosis of solid tumors. J Clin Oncol 21(13):2609–2615
24. Pantel K, Alix-Panabières C, Riethdorf S (2009) Cancer micrometastases. Nat Rev Clin Oncol 6(6):339–351
25. Pantel K, Brakenhoff RH (2004) Dissecting the metastatic cascade. Nat Rev Cancer 4(6):448–456
26. Ashworth TR (1869) A case of cancer in which cells similar to those in the tumours were seen in the blood after death. Aus Med J 14:146–149
27. Engell HC (1955) Cancer cells in the circulating blood; a clinical study on the occurrence of cancer cells in the peripheral blood and in venous blood draining the tumour area at operation. Acta Chir Scand Suppl 201:1–70
28. Salsbury AJ (1975) The significance of the circulating cancer cell. Cancer Treat Rev 2(1):55–72
29. Moss TJ, Sanders DG (1990) Detection of neuroblastoma cells in blood. J Clin Oncol 8(4):736–740

30. Leather AJ, Gallegos NC, Kocjan G, Savage F, Smales CS, Hu W, Boulos PB, Northover JM, Phillips RK (1993) Detection and enumeration of circulating tumour cells in colorectal cancer. Br J Surg 80(6):777–780
31. Brugger W, Bross KJ, Glatt M, Weber F, Mertelsmann R, Kanz L (1994) Mobilization of tumor cells and hematopoietic progenitor cells into peripheral blood of patients with solid tumors. Blood 83(3):636–640
32. Miller MC, Doyle GV, Terstappen LW (2010) Significance of circulating tumor cells detected by the cellsearch system in patients with metastatic breast colorectal and prostate cancer. J Oncol 2010:617421
33. Sun YF, Yang XR, Zhou J, Qiu SJ, Fan J, Xu Y (2011) Circulating tumor cells: advances in detection methods, biological issues, and clinical relevance. J Cancer Res Clin Oncol 137(8):1151–1173
34. Parkinson DR, Dracopoli N, Petty BG, Compton C, Cristofanilli M, Deisseroth A, Hayes DF, Kapke G, Kumar P, Lee JS, Liu MC, McCormack R, Mikulski S et al (2012) Considerations in the development of circulating tumor cell technology for clinical use. J Transl Med 10:138
35. King JD, Casavant BP, Lang JM (2014) Rapid translation of circulating tumor cell biomarkers into clinical practice: technology development, clinical needs and regulatory requirements. Lab Chip 14(1):24–31
36. Ignatiadis M, Lee M, Jeffrey SS (2015) Circulating tumor cells and circulating tumor DNA: challenges and opportunities on the path to clinical utility. Clin Cancer Res 21(21): 4786–4800
37. Cristofanilli M, Budd GT, Ellis MJ, Stopeck A, Matera J, Miller MC, Reuben JM, Doyle GV, Allard WJ, Terstappen LW, Hayes DF (2004) Circulating tumor cells, disease progression, and survival in metastatic breast cancer. N Engl J Med 351(8):781–791
38. Cohen SJ, Punt CJ, Iannotti N, Saidman BH, Sabbath KD, Gabrail NY, Picus J, Morse M, Mitchell E, Miller MC, Doyle GV, Tissing H, Terstappen LW et al (2008) Relationship of circulating tumor cells to tumor response, progression-free survival, and overall survival in patients with metastatic colorectal cancer. J Clin Oncol 26(19):3213–3221
39. Toss A, Mu Z, Fernandez S, Cristofanilli M (2014) CTC enumeration and characterization: moving toward personalized medicine. Ann Transl Med 2(11):108
40. Andree KC, van Dalum G, Terstappen LW (2016) Challenges in circulating tumor cell detection by the CellSearch system. Mol Oncol 10(3):395–407
41. Ignatiadis M, Rothé F, Chaboteaux C, Durbecq V, Rouas G, Criscitiello C, Metallo J, Kheddoumi N, Singhal SK, Michiels S, Veys I, Rossari J, Larsimont D et al (2011) HER2-positive circulating tumor cells in breast cancer. PLoS One 6(1):e15624
42. Meng S, Tripathy D, Shete S, Ashfaq R, Haley B, Perkins S, Beitsch P, Khan A, Euhus D, Osborne C, Frenkel E, Hoover S, Leitch M et al (2004) HER-2 gene amplification can be acquired as breast cancer progresses. Proc Natl Acad Sci U S A 101(25):9393–9398
43. Pestrin M, Bessi S, Puglisi F, Minisini AM, Masci G, Battelli N, Ravaioli A, Gianni L, Di Marsico R, Tondini C, Gori S, Coombes CR, Stebbing J et al (2012) Final results of a multicenter phase II clinical trial evaluating the activity of single-agent lapatinib in patients with HER2-negative metastatic breast cancer and HER2-positive circulating tumor cells. A proof-of-concept study. Breast Cancer Res Treat 134(1):283–289
44. Stebbing J, Payne R, Reise J, Frampton AE, Avery M, Woodley L, Di Leo A, Pestrin M, Krell J, Coombes RC (2013) The efficacy of lapatinib in metastatic breast cancer with HER2 non-amplified primary tumors and EGFR positive circulating tumor cells: a proof-of-concept study. PLoS One 8(5):e62543
45. Abdallah EA, Fanelli MF, Buim ME, Machado Netto MC, Gasparini Junior JL, Souza E, Silva V, Dettino AL, Mingues NB, Romero JV, Ocea LM, Rocha BM, Alves VS, Araújo DV et al (2015) Thymidylate synthase expression in circulating tumor cells: a new tool to predict 5-fluorouracil resistance in metastatic colorectal cancer patients. Int J Cancer 137(6):1397–1405
46. Miyamoto DT, Lee RJ, Stott SL, Ting DT, Wittner BS, Ulman M, Smas ME, Lord JB, Brannigan BW, Trautwein J, Bander NH, Wu CL, Sequist LV et al (2012) Androgen receptor

signaling in circulating tumor cells as a marker of hormonally responsive prostate cancer. Cancer Discov 2(11):995–1003

47. Maheswaran S, Sequist LV, Nagrath S, Ulkus L, Brannigan B, Collura CV, Inserra E, Diederichs S, Iafrate AJ, Bell DW, Digumarthy S, Muzikansky A, Irimia D et al (2008) Detection of mutations in EGFR in circulating lung-cancer cells. N Engl J Med 359(4):366–377

48. Deng G, Krishnakumar S, Powell AA, Zhang H, Mindrinos MN, Telli ML, Davis RW, Jeffrey SS (2014) Single cell mutational analysis of PIK3CA in circulating tumor cells and metastases in breast cancer reveals heterogeneity, discordance, and mutation persistence in cultured disseminated tumor cells from bone marrow. BMC Cancer 14:456

49. Pailler E, Adam J, Barthélémy A, Oulhen M, Auger N, Valent A, Borget I, Planchard D, Taylor M, André F, Soria JC, Vielh P, Besse B et al (2013) Detection of circulating tumor cells harboring a unique ALK rearrangement in ALK-positive non-small-cell lung cancer. J Clin Oncol 31(18):2273–2281

50. Fernandez SV, Bingham C, Fittipaldi P, Austin L, Palazzo J, Palmer G, Alpaugh K, Cristofanilli M (2014) TP53 mutations detected in circulating tumor cells present in the blood of metastatic triple negative breast cancer patients. Breast Cancer Res 16(5):445

51. Hou JM, Krebs MG, Lancashire L, Sloane R, Backen A, Swain RK, Priest LJ, Greystoke A, Zhou C, Morris K, Ward T, Blackhall FH, Dive C (2012) Clinical significance and molecular characteristics of circulating tumor cells and circulating tumor microemboli in patients with small-cell lung cancer. J Clin Oncol 30(5):525–532

52. Yu M, Bardia A, Wittner BS, Stott SL, Smas ME, Ting DT, Isakoff SJ, Ciciliano JC, Wells MN, Shah AM, Concannon KF, Donaldson MC, Sequist LV et al (2013) Circulating breast tumor cells exhibit dynamic changes in epithelial and mesenchymal composition. Science 339(6119):580–584

53. Aceto N, Bardia A, Miyamoto DT, Donaldson MC, Wittner BS, Spencer JA, Yu M, Pely A, Engstrom A, Zhu H, Brannigan BW, Kapur R, Stott SL et al (2014) Circulating tumor cell clusters are oligoclonal precursors of breast cancer metastasis. Cell 158(5):1110–1122

54. Alix-Panabières C, Pantel K (2014) Challenges in circulating tumour cell research. Nat Rev Cancer 14(9):623–631

55. Bidard FC, Fehm T, Ignatiadis M, Smerage JB, Alix-Panabières C, Janni W, Messina C, Paoletti C, Müller V, Hayes DF, Piccart M, Pierga JY (2013) Clinical application of circulating tumor cells in breast cancer: overview of the current interventional trials. Cancer Metastasis Rev 32(1–2):179–188

56. Mandel P, Metais P (1948) Les acides nucléiques du plasma sanguin chez l'homme. C R Seances Soc Biol Fil 142(3–4):241–243

57. Jahr S, Hentze H, Englisch S, Hardt D, Fackelmayer FO, Hesch RD, Knippers R (2001) DNA fragments in the blood plasma of cancer patients: quantitations and evidence for their origin from apoptotic and necrotic cells. Cancer Res 61(4):1659–1665

58. Stroun M, Lyautey J, Lederrey C, Mulcahy HE, Anker P (2001) Alu repeat sequences are present in increased proportions compared to a unique gene in plasma/serum DNA: evidence for a preferential release from viable cells? Ann N Y Acad Sci 945:258–264

59. Stroun M, Lyautey J, Lederrey C, Olson-Sand A, Anker P (2001) About the possible origin and mechanism of circulating DNA apoptosis and active DNA release. Clin Chim Acta 313(1–2):139–142

60. Diehl F, Schmidt K, Choti MA, Romans K, Goodman S, Li M, Thornton K, Agrawal N, Sokoll L, Szabo SA, Kinzler KW, Vogelstein B, Diaz LA Jr (2008) Circulating mutant DNA to assess tumor dynamics. Nat Med 14(9):985–990

61. Forshew T, Murtaza M, Parkinson C, Gale D, Tsui DW, Kaper F, Dawson SJ, Piskorz AM, Jimenez-Linan M, Bentley D, Hadfield J, May AP, Caldas C et al (2012) Noninvasive identification and monitoring of cancer mutations by targeted deep sequencing of plasma DNA. Sci Transl Med 4(136):136ra68

62. Shinozaki M, O'Day SJ, Kitago M, Amersi F, Kuo C, Kim J, Wang HJ, Hoon DS (2007) Utility of circulating B-RAF DNA mutation in serum for monitoring melanoma patients receiving biochemotherapy. Clin Cancer Res 13(7):2068–2074

63. Dawson SJ, Tsui DW, Murtaza M, Biggs H, Rueda OM, Chin SF, Dunning MJ, Gale D, Forshew T, Mahler-Araujo B, Rajan S, Humphray S, Becq J et al (2013) Analysis of circulating tumor DNA to monitor metastatic breast cancer. N Engl J Med 368(13):1199–1209
64. Diaz LA Jr, Bardelli A (2014) Liquid biopsies: genotyping circulating tumor DNA. J Clin Oncol 32(6):579–586
65. De Mattos-Arruda L, Weigelt B, Cortes J, Won HH, Ng CK, Nuciforo P, Bidard FC, Aura C, Saura C, Peg V, Piscuoglio S, Oliveira M, Smolders Y et al (2014) Capturing intra-tumor genetic heterogeneity by de novo mutation profiling of circulating cell-free tumor DNA: a proof-of-principle. Ann Oncol 25(9):1729–1735
66. Beaver JA, Jelovac D, Balukrishna S, Cochran RL, Croessmann S, Zabransky DJ, Wong HY, Valda Toro P, Cidado J, Blair BG, Chu D, Burns T, Higgins MJ et al (2014) Detection of cancer DNA in plasma of patients with early-stage breast cancer. Clin Cancer Res 20(10): 2643–2650
67. Kinugasa H, Nouso K, Miyahara K, Morimoto Y, Dohi C, Tsutsumi K, Kato H, Matsubara T, Okada H, Yamamoto K (2015) Detection of K-ras gene mutation by liquid biopsy in patients with pancreatic cancer. Cancer 121(13):2271–2280
68. Bettegowda C, Sausen M, Leary RJ, Kinde I, Wang Y, Agrawal N, Bartlett BR, Wang H, Luber B, Alani RM, Antonarakis ES, Azad NS, Bardelli A et al (2014) Detection of circulating tumor DNA in early- and late-stage human malignancies. Sci Transl Med 6(224):224ra24
69. Higgins MJ, Jelovac D, Barnathan E, Blair B, Slater S, Powers P, Zorzi J, Jeter SC, Oliver GR, Fetting J, Emens L, Riley C, Stearns V et al (2012) Detection of tumor PIK3CA status in metastatic breast cancer using peripheral blood. Clin Cancer Res 18(12):3462–3469
70. Rothé F, Laes JF, Lambrechts D, Smeets D, Vincent D, Maetens M, Fumagalli D, Michiels S, Drisis S, Moerman C, Detiffe JP, Larsimont D, Awada A et al (2014) Plasma circulating tumor DNA as an alternative to metastatic biopsies for mutational analysis in breast cancer. Ann Oncol 25(10):1959–1965
71. Madic J, Kiialainen A, Bidard FC, Birzele F, Ramey G, Leroy Q, Rio Frio T, Vaucher I, Raynal V, Bernard V, Lermine A, Clausen I, Giroud N et al (2015) Circulating tumor DNA and circulating tumor cells in metastatic triple negative breast cancer patients. Int J Cancer 136(9):2158–2165
72. Thierry AR, Mouliere F, El Messaoudi S, Mollevi C, Lopez-Crapez E, Rolet F, Gillet B, Gongora C, Dechelotte P, Robert B, Del Rio M, Lamy PJ, Bibeau F et al (2014) Clinical validation of the detection of KRAS and BRAF mutations from circulating tumor DNA. Nat Med 20(4):430–435
73. Punnoose EA, Atwal S, Liu W, Raja R, Fine BM, Hughes BG, Hicks RJ, Hampton GM, Amler LC, Pirzkall A, Lackner MR (2012) Evaluation of circulating tumor cells and circulating tumor DNA in non-small cell lung cancer: association with clinical endpoints in a phase II clinical trial of pertuzumab and erlotinib. Clin Cancer Res 18(8):2391–2401
74. Al-Nedawi K, Meehan B, Micallef J, Lhotak V, May L, Guha A, Rak J (2008) Intercellular transfer of the oncogenic receptor EGFRvIII by microvesicles derived from tumour cells. Nat Cell Biol 10(5):619–624
75. Balaj L, Lessard R, Dai L, Cho YJ, Pomeroy SL, Breakefield XO, Skog J (2011) Tumour microvesicles contain retrotransposon elements and amplified oncogene sequences. Nat Commun 2:180
76. Miranda KC, Bond DT, McKee M, Skog J, Păunescu TG, Da Silva N, Brown D, Russo LM (2010) Nucleic acids within urinary exosomes/microvesicles are potential biomarkers for renal disease. Kidney Int 78(2):191–199
77. Ratajczak J, Wysoczynski M, Hayek F, Janowska-Wieczorek A, Ratajczak MZ (2006) Membrane-derived microvesicles: important and underappreciated mediators of cell-to-cell communication. Leukemia 20(9):1487–1495 Epub 2006 Jul 20
78. Skog J, Würdinger T, van Rijn S, Meijer DH, Gainche L, Sena-Esteves M, Curry WT Jr, Carter BS, Krichevsky AM, Breakefield XO (2008) Glioblastoma microvesicles transport RNA and proteins that promote tumour growth and provide diagnostic biomarkers. Nat Cell Biol 10(12):1470–1476

79. Thakur BK, Zhang H, Becker A, Matei I, Huang Y, Costa-Silva B, Zheng Y, Hoshino A, Brazier H, Xiang J, Williams C, Rodriguez-Barrueco R, Silva JM et al (2014) Double-stranded DNA in exosomes: a novel biomarker in cancer detection. Cell Res 24(6):766–769
80. Nilsson J, Skog J, Nordstrand A, Baranov V, Mincheva-Nilsson L, Breakefield XO, Widmark A (2009) Prostate cancer-derived urine exosomes: a novel approach to biomarkers for prostate cancer. Br J Cancer 100(10):1603–1607
81. Chen WW, Balaj L, Liau LM, Samuels ML, Kotsopoulos SK, Maguire CA, Loguidice L, Soto H, Garrett M, Zhu LD, Sivaraman S, Chen C, Wong ET et al (2013) BEAMing and droplet digital PCR analysis of mutant IDH1 mRNA in glioma patient serum and cerebrospinal fluid extracellular vesicles. Mol Ther Nucleic Acids 2:e109
82. Peinado H, Alečković M, Lavotshkin S, Matei I, Costa-Silva B, Moreno-Bueno G, Hergueta-Redondo M, Williams C, García-Santos G, Ghajar C, Nitadori-Hoshino A, Hoffman C et al (2012) Melanoma exosomes educate bone marrow progenitor cells toward a pro-metastatic phenotype through MET. Nat Med 18(6):883–891
83. Whiteside TL (2013) Immune modulation of T-cell and NK (natural killer) cell activities by TEXs (tumour-derived exosomes). Biochem Soc Trans 41(1):245–251
84. Yáñez-Mó M, Siljander PR, Andreu Z, Zavec AB, Borràs FE, Buzas EI, Buzas K, Casal E, Cappello F, Carvalho J, Colás E, Cordeiro-da Silva A, Fais S et al (2015) Biological properties of extracellular vesicles and their physiological functions. J Extracell Vesicles 4:27066

Chapter 2
Circulating Tumour Cells in Primary Disease: The Seed for Metastasis

Noam Falbel Pondé and Michail Ignatiadis

Abstract Metastatic dissemination is the most common cause of death in cancer patients. Traditionally, dissemination has been considered a late event; however it has been suggested that at least in some tumours, cells might leave the primary lesion early in its development. To escape from the primary, tumour cells undergo total or partial epithelial to mesenchymal transition (EMT), become able to unmoor from surrounding epithelial cells and reach the bloodstream. Alone or in groups (clusters), these circulating tumour cells will use their phenotypical flexibility, including properties associated with EMT, stemness, resistance to anoikis and dormancy to survive in the bloodstream, reach, invade and colonise distant organs. In recent years, these cells, which can be detected in the blood or in the bone marrow in the early disease setting, have been studied as prognostic markers as well as a potential source of dynamic information regarding tumour characteristics to guide treatment decisions. Ongoing clinical trials are evaluating the clinical utility of circulating tumour cells.

Keywords Circulating tumour cells • Cell clusters • Epithelial-mesenchymal transition • Dormancy • Reseeding • Phenotypical flexibility • Stemness • Liquid biopsy • Heterogeneity • HER2 status discordance

Introduction

Despite the advances in the treatment of breast cancer (BC) achieved in the last 30 years, development of metastatic disease is still a major cause of death for women diagnosed with BC [1]. Metastasis formation is a highly inefficient process in which tumour cells leave the primary tumour, enter the bloodstream, invade other organs and colonise them, forming secondary tumours (metastasis) [2–4]. Technological advances have allowed the detection of tumour cells circulating in the bloodstream—called circulating tumour cells (CTCs)—and of tumour cells that have invaded other organs called disseminated tumour cells (DTCs) [5–7].

N.F. Pondé • M. Ignatiadis (✉)
Department of Medical Oncology, Institut Jules Bordet,
Boulevard de Waterloo, 121, Brussels 1000, Belgium
e-mail: noam.ponde@bordet.be; michail.ignatiadis@bordet.be

© Springer International Publishing AG 2017
M. Cristofanilli (ed.), *Liquid Biopsies in Solid Tumors*, Cancer Drug Discovery and Development, DOI 10.1007/978-3-319-50956-3_2

Both CTCs and DTCs have been the focus of intense translational research in the last 20 years. Interest in them is driven by the insights they can provide into the underpinnings of the process of cancer dissemination, leading possibly to new therapeutic targets, as well as how they may inform us on the dynamic changes in tumour genotype and phenotype that occur during treatment [6, 8, 9].

In this chapter, we provide a review of the findings from CTC research that have led to a better understanding of the dissemination process with special emphasis on BC. We focus on the contributions of CTC research to the key concepts of epithelial to mesenchymal transition (EMT), stemness, dormancy and self-seeding, as well as the potential role of CTC clusters in dissemination. Finally, we discuss studies on the prognostic significance of CTCs/DTCs and on characterisation of these cells and ongoing interventional trials testing CTCs as tools to improve outcome of patients with early BC.

Circulating Tumour Cells and the Biology of Metastasis

Definition of Circulating Tumour Cells

CTCs were first detected in BC patients 150 years ago [10] and are shed by the primary tumour during the dissemination process. They are rare events detected in the bloodstream (1 for every $10^6/10^7$ mononuclear cells). CTCs can leave the primary tumour either alone (single CTCs) or in clusters with other tumour cells and/ or surrounding stromal cells and matrix (respectively, homotypic or heterotypic CTC clusters, Fig. 2.1) [6, 7, 11]. Though several aspects of CTC/DTC biology are not entirely understood, one characteristic of these cells is phenotypical plasticity, i.e. the ability to undergo phenotypic changes in order to survive [7, 12–14].

Models of Metastatic Progression

Models of metastatic progression have evolved from the nineteenth century onwards and are generally based on the assumption that cells harbouring genetic or epigenetic alterations evolve within a Darwinian framework, acquiring progressively the malignant phenotype [15]. In BC specifically the original Halstedian model assumed progression in a local, centrifugal fashion before invasion of distant organs, stressing as a consequence local versus systemic therapeutic approaches [16, 17]. Over time, with increasing knowledge on tumour biology including studies on CTC/DTCs, our understanding has evolved significantly and today emphasizes the systemic nature of BC [3, 18].

The Linear and Parallel Progression Models

The model of linear progression from preinvasive to invasive and to metastatic tumour assumes that metastasis results from pre-existing highly metastatic rare cells within the primary tumour [19]. This model is supported by the clinical observation

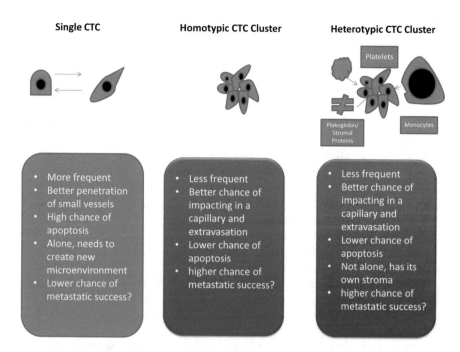

Fig. 2.1 Comparison between single CTC, homotypic clusters and heterotypic clusters

that larger tumours tend to be more often metastatic at presentation or to recur more frequently post-curative treatment than smaller tumours and is the basis for current screening and treatment guidelines [20, 21]. Though the linear model emphasises the systemic nature of cancer [3], CTCs and DTCs are deemed to be late events, the product of successive generations of cells undergoing natural selection within the primary tumour, acquiring most if not all of capabilities necessary to successfully disseminate and eventually leaving the primary to form distant metastasis [19, 22].

However, the linear model alone does not adequately explain a number of clinical scenarios. Though patients with T2–4 or N-positive BC have a higher chance of developing local or distant recurrences, still, 4% of patients with tumours smaller than 1 cm will die from cancer in 10 years [23]. Moreover, evidence from clinical studies on CTCs/DTCs and from studies using murine models suggests that dissemination may start earlier than previously thought [18, 24, 25].

In one study by Banis and colleagues, 16% out of 404 patients with ductal carcinoma in situ (DCIS) scheduled to undergo surgery had detectable DTCs in the BM. No correlation with lymph node positivity or survival was found [26]. The same group as well as other investigators have found similar results in smaller studies of patients with DCIS or microinvasive disease [27, 28]. In the landmark meta-analysis published in 2005 with a total of 4703 patients, 25.2% of patients with T1 tumours had detectable DTCs in the BM [29]. Indirect clinical evidence for early dissemination has also been provided by studies on the adverse prognostic value of

CTC detection in patients with early breast cancer [30, 31]. We have detected CTCs in the bloodstream of 9% (6/73) of women with DCIS/LCIS [32].

Beyond the above clinical studies, there is evidence from preclinical studies that dissemination might occur early on during the process of metastasis.

Podsypanina and colleagues showed that non-cancerous murine mammary cells injected into the bloodstream can survive inside lung tissue. These cells can undergo malignant transformation forming lung metastasis completely independently from the existence of a primary tumour [33].

Another group studied the development of metastasis before the appearance of primary tumour in a model of BC in mice that are carriers of the polyoma virus middle T oncogene. The development of primary BC in these mice happened in stages—first hyperplasia around 26 days after birth, followed by solid masses developed at around 60 days and finally invasive tumours by 116 days. In contrast, cultures of lung tissue showed cells capable of forming tumour colonies at day 26. These cells were morphologically similar to mammary cancer cells and expressed cancer stem cell (CSC) markers CD44 and Sca1 [34].

In a landmark study using mice that have a constitutionally activated human epidermal growth factor receptor 2 (HER2) gene, Hüsemann and colleagues showed that DTCs can be detected in the bone marrow of mice during the preinvasive phase of tumour progression [24]. The mice develop mammary hyperplasia between weeks 7 and 9, in situ lesions by 14–18 and overtly invasive disease by 23–30 weeks. In the BM, DTCs were already detectable in some cases as early as week 4. Interestingly, as primaries grew in size, the number of DTCs as well as the number of genetic alterations in these cells remained fairly stable.

Taken together, these data suggest that cells might leave the primary tumour early during tumour development and evolve in parallel with cells in the primary tumour (parallel progression model). This model implies genomic heterogeneity between primary tumour and distant metastasis, since there is a parallel evolution in the primary and distant site. This model, if true, challenges our capacity to infer genomic profiles for micrometastatic disease based on the analyses of the primary tumour and might at least partly explain why some patients with early BC relapse and die despite adjuvant systemic treatment. On the other hand, the fact that adjuvant treatment based on primary tumour characteristics is effective in reducing relapses and the existence of effective primary tumour-based gene signatures that predict the risk of distant relapse [35] suggests that the parallel progression model alone cannot explain a significant proportion of BC cases.

Tumour Self-Seeding

Self-seeding is another complementary hypothesis that has been supported by recent experimental evidence, which postulates that CTCs and DTCs, now "veterans" of the hard evolutionary struggle of invasion, survival in the bloodstream and colonisation of distant organs, return to the primary tumour, an environment likely to prove more welcoming to them [36–38].

The pivotal studies conducted by Kim and colleagues were designed to evaluate this intriguing hypothesis [39]. In a murine model, the investigators injected two mammary glands with a metastatic BC cell line, one marked with GFP-luciferase (donor) and another without (recipient). After 60 days recipient tumours had extensive seeding by donor cells (up to a quarter of total mass). In a further study the same group of researchers showed that this 'homing" effect is possibly achieved through chemo-attractants such as interleukin-6 and interleukin-8. Interestingly, the rate of growth in the seeded primary was accelerated mainly by increased number of cells through a paracrine effect, suggesting that self-seeding can induce increased growth in the primary [39].

Zhang and colleagues in a series of experiments using an osteosarcoma murine model encountered very similar results [40]. The hypothesis that interleukin signalling mediates self-seeding has been further strengthened by a recent publication by the same group showing that suppression of IL-6 halts self-seeding [41].

Apart from the above preclinical studies, indirect evidence supporting the hypothesis of self-seeding has been provided by a clinical study in which 3072 patients undergoing surgery for BC were submitted to a BM biopsy. 732 (24%) had DTCs, 139 patients experienced local recurrence and 48 of these (35%) were DTC positive. Being DTC positive was significantly associated with a higher risk of local recurrence [42], suggesting that DTCs can influence local recurrence.

Steps in the Invasive: Metastatic Cascade

The success of a CTC/DTC is measured by its capacity in actually generating metastasis. In order to achieve this, a complex series of events must take place called the invasive-metastatic cascade. This process involves cancer cells as well as multiple other actors and can be divided into several steps [3, 43].

Local Invasion and Intravasation

In epithelial tumours, cells will face severe challenges before they are able to disseminate. To reach the bloodstream, cancer cells must first break through the barrier formed by surrounding cells, underlying stroma and endothelial cells. There is no single path to tissue invasion, with multiple mechanisms both active and passive coming into play to result either in individual invasion or collective invasion and intravasation, mirroring the two forms in which CTCs may be detected—single or clustered [43, 44]. In both, however, the process of EMT is fundamental.

Epithelial-Mesenchymal Transition

Epithelial cells share characteristics that make them well adapted to their function of forming cell barriers. Apical-basal polarity and tight cell-to-cell binding through desmosomes and between cell and basal layer through hemidesmosomes allow for their organisation into highly structured sheets of cells, such as in the skin or the intra-ductal epithelium of the breast [45]. However, during physiological situations such as organogenesis and wound healing, epithelial cells must be able to move alone and in groups as well as to change shape, abilities more often associated with mesenchymal cells [46]. This process of phenotypic plasticity through which epithelial cells lose their epithelial characteristics and acquire those of mesenchymal cells is named epithelial-mesenchymal transition (EMT). EMT is driven by cell-to-cell communication through various cytokines—such as between epithelial cells and cancer-associated fibroblasts or macrophages. This interaction leads to activation of pathways such as transforming growth factor beta (TGFbeta), epidermal growth factor (EGF) and hepatocyte growth factor (HGF) signalling pathways [47, 48], by inducing one of the EMT-associated transcription factors, including TWIST1, SNAI1 or SLUG [49]. To test the importance of cytokine milieu produced by activated monocytes (MCs) in inducing EMT, Cohen and colleagues exposed in vitro cell lines from both inflammatory BC and non-inflammatory BC to activated MCs, with results showing increased cellular motility as well as a morphological and protein expression shift towards a mesenchymal phenotype.

For a cancer cell seeking to leave the primary tumour (or preinvasive lesion) and to cross the endothelium to reach the intravascular space [50], EMT is instrumental [13, 51]. Complete EMT (where all epithelial characteristics are lost) can lead to individual invasion. The cell loses traditional epithelial polarity and proteins (E-cadherin, plakoglobin and integrins) that form the attachment organelles, freeing it to enter conjunctive tissue underneath. During this process it acquires one of the two possible phenotypes:

1. A mesenchymal-like shape with lamellipodia and filopodia granting ability to adhere to the extracellular matrix (ECM) through N-cadherin: These cells produce enzymes such as the metalloproteinases (MMP) that play several key roles in BC progression, including the degradation of the ECM, of cell-to-cell junctions, stimulation of cell motility and interestingly the induction of EMT directly and indirectly (by influencing surrounding cancer-associated cells) [52, 53]. Thus, it can be said of these cells that through intercellular communication they become true "microenvironment engineers" with the goal of constructing the environment that maximises their chance of invasion [54].

2. Amoeboid, with round-shaped cells that can pass through gaps formed by other cells in the ECM (macrophages, for instance): It is MMP independent, and tightly regulated through interplay between RHO kinase and the GTPase RAC [55]. The relevance of this mode of movement in vivo is still controversial since artificial models of ECM microenvironment may not be accurate, possibly allowing for cellular motility that would not be possible in vivo [56, 57], leading some experts to challenge the invasive potential of this phenotype.

Recent studies demonstrate the existence of populations of CTCs that express markers for EMT, and are not detected through traditional EpCAM-based methods [58, 59]. Their study has been expanded by the increasing perception of their special clinical and biological relevance. Other mesenchymal markers are being used to detect them, such as vimentin, Twist and N-cadherin [60].

In a recent study in 149 patients with early BC, Cierna and colleagues sought to investigate the presence of CTCs with EMT markers, as well as their correlation with MMP1 in tumour tissue and stroma [61]. CTCs with epithelial markers were present in 8.7% of patients and CTCs with epithelial-mesenchymal transition (EMT) markers in 13.4% of patients. Patients with CTC/EMT in peripheral blood had significantly increased expression of MMP1 in tumour cells and tumour-associated stroma ($p = 0.05$) than those of patients without CTC/EMT. MMP1 expression was associated with tumour features such as high grade or high proliferation (Ki 67 > 20%), both markers of worse prognosis.

In an animal model of CTC EMT composed of mice bearing metastatic BC grafts from human cancer, Gorges and colleagues were able to detect CTCs with EMT markers that an EpCAM-based method could not detect [58]. To test the theory that cells injected into the bloodstream of a mouse would down-regulate EpCAM (a phenomenon used here as a surrogate marker for EMT), they injected tumour cells that expressed epithelial markers, and looked for them for 30 min to 4 h after injection. CTCs showed morphological changes and down-regulated EpCAM within 30 min from injection. Some cells, however, presented expression patterns that were mixed. The above results suggest that the regulation of phenotypic changes in tumour cells is a dynamic process [58].

Partial EMT, a process that leads to cells with mixed epithelial-mesenchymal features, might be the most efficient pathway to dissemination [57]. While complete EMT leads more likely to the shedding of single cells, in partial EMT clumps or clusters of between 2 and 50 cells will be shed together with parts of their microenvironment, including cancer-associated cells and ECM, possibly leading to survival and colonisation advantages [11, 57, 62, 63].

To reach the bloodstream cells must breach blood vessels, a step facilitated by tumour stimulation of the formation of new vessels that are tortuous and "leaky". The MMPs that participate in previous steps are also important in this process of formation of new vessels and constant remodelling [64].

Survival in the Circulation and Extravasation

Dissemination is an inefficient process, and most CTCs will not successfully form metastasis [65]. In practice, most CTCs detected are apoptotic [66]. Different phenomena account for this high failure rate and are connected to challenges the CTC will face in the bloodstream.

Single Circulating Tumour Cells

Once in the bloodstream, different mechanisms can lead to the apoptosis of singe CTCs such as anoikis and the shear stress exerted by the blood current. The high failure rate at this phase is well exemplified by a study by Tarin and colleagues performed in 1984 on 15 cancer patients with neoplastic ascites. Peritoneovenous shunts were placed to alleviate ascites and as a consequence a high number of tumour cells were injected into the circulation. Surprisingly, very few patients went on to develop solid metastasis in the following months or even years, in one case [67].

Anoikis can be defined as apoptosis induced by disconnection from the ECM and from surrounding cells; it seems to be a built-in safeguard against unmoored epithelial cells that can disrupt tissue cohesion. It is therefore a process that all successful tumour cells must evade to survive. Many of the signalling pathways harnessed for increased proliferation in cancer can confer resistance to anoikis, such as EGFR. More significantly, EMT (total or partial) also can confer resistance to it [7, 68].

The shear stress produced by circulation of blood is recognised as being capable of inducing phenotypic changes in endothelial cells that are fundamental to normal vessel function but also to impact the dissemination process [69, 70]. Recent experiments in colon and prostate cancer CTCs suggest that shear force can induce apoptosis via TRAIL in time (duration of shear stress) and dose (strength of shear stress) dependent fashion [71]. This observation may have clinical implication as TRAIL receptor inducers are now in phase I and II testing [72].

Finally, the immune system plays a role likely by clearing cells through natural killer lymphocytes as well as other immune cells. As shown by an experiment by Steinert and colleagues in colon cancer CTCs adaptive pressure caused by immune cells gives rise to CTCs with a CD47 hyper-expressing phenotype that inhibits the activity of immune cells [73].

Clustered Circulating Tumour Cells

The existence of CTC clusters has in the past been used, among other arguments, to question the in vivo relevance of EMT, but, as we have previously discussed, they are not incompatible. Clusters allow for higher ability to survive, resistance to anoikis and higher chance of adhering at secondary sites [7, 74]. Recent evidence suggests that clusters are more capable to lead to successful colonisation compared to single CTCs [11].

CTC clusters are widely present in different epithelial tumours, and can potentially be formed through cells leaving the tumour together or aggregating in the bloodstream [75]. One experiment in an immunodeficient mice model, using a cell line of lung metastatic cells engineered to express either green fluorescent protein or m-cherry in a 1:1 ratio, was conducted by Aceto and colleagues. Cells were injected into the fat pads of mice. Search for CTCs in their blood once overt tumours were present at the injection site uncovered both clustered (2.6%) and single cells (97.4%). Ninety-one percent of the clusters were positive for both protein markers. Nine percent of clusters were of single origin, and none of the single-origin clusters were larger than three cells (suggesting that clusters are not the product of intravessel proliferation of one cell). An examination of the mice's lungs showed that 53% of metastases were of dual origin (and therefore were the product of clusters) and 47% of single origin. This suggests that while single CTCs are more common, clusters successfully form metastasis 50 times more often. In a second experiment, the same group investigated the issue of the origin of clusters—formation by random aggregation in the bloodstream versus group exit from the primary. The same differently marked cells were injected, this time in different fat pads. A total of 96% of resulting clusters were of single colour, suggesting that intravascular formation of a cluster is a minor phenomenon. Another provocative result of this experiment came from the analysis of the primary. Up to 5% of the cells in each primary carried the opposite colour tag, suggesting that cells can invade the primary lesion (self-seeding). Further experiments by the same authors showed that clusters displayed higher resistance to apoptosis and faster clearance from blood—probably secondary to capillary entrapment that may favour metastasisation. In the blood of ten patients with metastatic BC the same authors were able to define that the gene encoding the protein plakoglobin is highly overexpressed in clusters [11].

The enhanced ability of CTC clusters to form metastasis has been corroborated by three recently published studies. In a cohort of 115 patients, single CTCs and clusters were detected in 36 (31.3%) and 20 (17.4%) of patients, respectively. Though both findings predicted worse prognosis, it was in patients where both were present that the risk of progression was the highest. In another study, in an advanced triple-negative breast cancer population, CTCs (both single and clustered) were correlated with worse prognosis. Interestingly cells detected in clusters had a much lower chance of being apoptotic [76]. In lung cancer one study reported similar findings on cluster cell apoptosis, as well as, significantly, that clusters expressed mesenchymal markers in a heterogeneous manner (vimentin and E-cadherin), compatible with different cells undergoing EMT to different degrees [77].

Plakoglobin is one of the molecular components of the cell-to-cell junctures called desmosomes and plays a vital role in maintaining the cohesiveness of CTC clusters. Suppression of plakoglobin expression has been suggested to inhibit the formation of clusters and metastasisation [11]. This result nicely complements work from Holen and colleagues on the role of plakoglobin in invasion. Blocking plakoglobin expression led, in vitro, to reduced adhesion between cells and enhanced invasion through an artificial model of the basement membrane. In vivo suppression led to greater growth of the primary, but no formation of metastasis, despite evidence of more than a 2.5-fold increase in CTCs [78].

What hypothesis can be drawn from the above studies? It seems that clusters of cells that undergo partial EMT and thus keep enough adhesive capabilities to maintain cohesion and even stroma inside the bloodstream can better survive in the bloodstream [11, 62, 79]. These cells may be more adept at initiating metastasis. Associating in the bloodstream with platelets and other cells remains as important as it was in invasion or as it will be during colonisation [80]. The paradoxical role of plakoglobin, however, on the one hand during invasion and exit from primary acting as a barrier, and then as an essential component for effective dissemination, shows that, for CTCs, increased metastatic potential may be associated not only with numbers, but also with phenotypical flexibility, upregulating and downregulating pathways as their expression becomes necessary or deleterious. For extravasation, as well as for other steps in the metastatic cascade, this flexibility is associated with the ability to disrupt normal micro-vessel permeability and is mediated via the secretion of paracrine factors such as angiopoietins and MMPs [3].

Formation of Metastasis

Once extravasation has occurred tumour cells will face the challenge of colonisation. To do so successfully a few key abilities are vital, including the ability to influence the new microenvironment as well as related different cellular states, such as dormancy and stemness.

Disseminated Tumour Cells in the Bone Marrow

The invasion of the BM in BC is a long established fact. As a model of metastatic invasion of tissues and organs, BM is highly valuable, though with the caveat that the application to the clinic is hampered by the fact that BM aspiration is not a routine part of clinical practice in BC [81].

As previously discussed, studies suggest that BM DTCs are present early on during BC development. However, it seems that not all DTCs are capable of colonisation, as is shown by Braun and colleagues in a combined analysis of 4703 BC patients with detectable DTCs with early or locally advanced disease. Of these, despite DTCs being a negative prognostic factor for this cohort, after 10 years <50% had recurred [29].

The crucial bottleneck in this step is the ability to influence a foreign microenvironment. A number of studies have shown that specific genetic signatures facilitate the colonisation by DTCs of different organs and are likely associated with the capacity of DTCs to effectively communicate with surrounding cells in order to achieve colonisation [3]. When unable to do so DTCs may be eliminated or enter a quiescent state called dormancy.

Dormancy

Dormancy is a reversible state of mitotic arrest (or alternatively very slow rate of mitosis) first defined in the 1940–1950s [82]. It allows DTCs to endure unfavourable environments so that they can be able to colonise at a later stage. From a clinical standpoint, it is at the heart of resistance to adjuvant therapy and of late recurrences in BC [12, 14, 83].

There remains a large area of uncertainty regarding the mechanisms that induce dormancy and especially that cause reactivation from dormancy. Dormancy has been suggested to be the results of microenvironmental factors associated with limited angiogenesis and active immune response. Altered signalling through pathways such as the RAS-MEK-ERK/MAPK and PI(3)K/AKT can also induce dormancy.

Therefore, it is possible that dormancy may be a programmed reaction by a DTC installed into a microenvironment in which it cannot thrive, likely due to ineffective communication with surrounding cells [84].

Some interesting experiments on CTC/DTCs have shed some light into this phenomenon. In a model of dormancy, Naumov and colleagues used two different murine BC DTC lines, one slowly metastatic, with large numbers of dormant cells, and another rapidly disseminating, with a small number of dormant cells. Adriamycin treatment was not effective in the dormant subgroups of both cell lines, suggesting that dormancy is a mechanism of adjuvant chemotherapy resistance in BC. This finding correlates with clinical scenarios in triple-negative breast cancer (TNBC) and ER-positive BC during post-treatment follow-up. TNBC is more aggressive and highly responsive to chemotherapy and seldom recurs after 5 years, suggesting (following the above model) a low ratio of dormant cells. In ER-positive tumours, specially luminal A, there is low sensitivity to chemotherapy and a tendency towards late relapses, bespeaking of a high number of dormant cells [85, 86].

In one study investigating the angiogenic phenotype, Rogers and colleagues showed that in vitro, a cell line of liposarcoma that was originally not capable of angiogenesis formed small tumours, but at around 125 days acquired the capacity of producing larger vessels (angiogenic switch), going on thereafter to rapidly proliferate. However, in each consecutive cell generation, 6–8% of new cells reverted to the non-angiogenic dormant state. This underscores that, like EMT/MET, dormancy is a state of cancer cells and that cancer cells can go in and out, as needed [87].

In a study with 36 patients 7 years post-mastectomy, Meng and colleagues showed that 13 (36%) had detectable CTCs, up to 22 years after treatment. CTC clearance is approximately 1–2.4 h, so it is reasonable to assume that the origin of these cells is in slowly replicating/dormant groups of DTCs where the number of divisions is matched by the number of cells that undergo apoptosis or are shed [88].

Stemness

Cancer stem cell (CSC) theory, also called tumour-initiating cell theory, postulates that a subgroup among cancer cells is responsible for the formation of metastasis. Since earlier discussed studies show that CTCs when injected into fat pads lead to formation of local tumours, it is reasonable to assume that a subpopulation of CTCs and DTCs have properties of tumour-initiating cells. The main characteristics of these cells are their ability for self-renewal and for formation of non-CSC progeny [89], as well as their resistance to chemotherapy. At least in some instances, CSC may not be a separate category of cells, but indeed a transient state that can be activated and deactivated, and that is closely connected to EMT [90]. There are several studies in BC, showing that significant portions of CTCs and DTCs express CSC markers.

Aktas and colleagues analysed blood samples from 39 patients with BC and showed that 80% of patients with CTCs overexpressed EMT markers or the CSC marker ALDH1 [91]. In another study, Giordano and colleagues studied samples from 29 women with MBC, and found a correlation between CTCs with EMT markers and CSC markers [92]. This association between EMT and stemness was investigated in depth by Mani et al., in a pivotal series of experiments [93]. Murine immortalised cells that were previously not able to form tumours were stimulated to undergo EMT. The resulting cells had the expected morphological and protein expression patterns, and were also largely CD44^{high}/CD24^{low}, a phenotype strongly associated with CSC. These cells were able to form mammospheres (a standard in vitro surrogate for tumour-forming potential). Furthermore, analyses of these mammospheres showed that only 4–6% of cells were capable of forming new ones. In another experiment, a population of CSC was analysed, looking for EMT markers. Results showed that these cells expressed EMT-related genes at levels similar to CTCs that had undergone EMT [93]. One study of 66 patients with early BC found that 48.6% of patients had DTCs and that 43% of detected DTCs had stem cell-like phenotype [94]. Patients with TNBC had a higher chance of having DTCs with stem cell-like phenotype in the BM [94]. Multiple other studies have confirmed that CTCs with EMT and stem cell-like markers can be found in the bloodstream of BC patients [95, 96]. Moreover, bone marrow DTCs with stem cell-like phenotype have shown to be an unfavourable prognostic marker in BC [97].

Taken together these results show that a subpopulation of CTCs and DTCs express stem cell-like markers, and that stemness may be a state associated with EMT that can be acquired by tumour cells.

Clinical Applications of Circulating Tumour Cells

The clinical potential of CTCs/DTCs has been intensively studied in the last 15 years [98] and multiple detection methods are available, that have been recently summarised [6, 99]. CTCs in the early setting can be used (Fig. 2.2):

1. As screening tools
2. As prognostic factors
3. For identifying therapeutic targets
4. For monitoring response to treatment

These applications may be achieved via enumeration or characterisation of CTCs at the deoxyribonucleic acid (DNA), ribonucleic acid (RNA) and protein levels.

Circulating Tumour Cells as Prognostic Factors

In early BC a large number of studies have demonstrated the adverse prognostic value of CTC/DTC detection (Table 2.1) [30, 31, 100–109, 112–124, 126].

Zhang and colleagues have performed a meta-analysis of both early disease and metastatic trials, totalling 49 studies and 6825 patients [129]. In early disease CTC detection was associated with worse DFS and OS (HR 2.86 and 2.78, respectively).

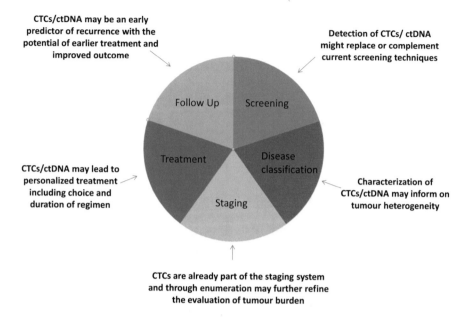

CTCs/ctDNA may be an early predictor of recurrence with the potential of earlier treatment and improved outcome

Detection of CTCs/ ctDNA might replace or complement current screening techniques

CTCs/ctDNA may lead to personalized treatment including choice and duration of regimen

Characterization of CTCs/ctDNA may inform on tumour heterogeneity

CTCs are already part of the staging system and through enumeration may further refine the evaluation of tumour burden

Fig. 2.2 Potential clinical applications of CTCs/ctDNA

In a recently published pooled analysis of individual data from 3173 patients with early BC, Janni and colleagues detected CTCs in 20.2% of the patients. Detection of CTCs was an independent prognostic factor for DFS, distant disease-free survival (DDFS) and OS. Patients with detectable CTCs had more often larger tumours, greater lymph node involvement and a higher tumour grade [126].

In the largest study to date in early breast cancer, Rack and colleagues evaluated retrospectively 1492 pre- and post-adjuvant chemotherapy. Before chemotherapy 21.5% were CTC positive and after chemotherapy 22.4%. The presence of CTCs was significantly correlated with worse DFS and OS. Interestingly a higher number of detectable CTCs (more than 5 per 30 mL of blood) determined worse outcomes [123]. Another, smaller prospective study on 302 patients with 24% positive samples had similar results [121].

This data as well as smaller studies (Table 2.1) and data on DTCs in the same setting [29] have led to a change in BC staging, with the creation of the cM0(i+) category, though this is seldom used in clinical practice at this point in time [98].

Circulating Tumour Cell Characterisation

Characterisation studies with CTCs hold the potential of more precise guidance to treatment than simple enumeration. Via the investigation of different markers CTC subpopulations may be identified that determine a worse outcome or that may

Table 2.1 Clinical studies with CTCs in early breast cancer

Author	Detection method	Number of patients	Timing	Detection rate	Prognostic	Marker
Stathopoulos et al. [100]	RT-PCR	111	Pre- and post-chemotherapy	36%	No	CK-19 mRNA
Gaforio et al. [101][a]	ICC	92	Pre-chemotherapy	62%	PFS and OS	CK
Xenidis et al. [102]	RT-PCR	161	Post chemotherapy	27.3	RFS	CK-19 mRNA
Giatromanolaki et al. [103]	RT-PCR	100	Pre-chemotherapy	33%	RFS	CK-19 mRNA
Pierga et al. [104][a]	ICC	114	Post-chemotherapy	24.5%	No	CKs 8, 18, 19
Masuda et al. [105]	RT-PCR	206	Pre-chemotherapy	18%	RFS	CK-7
Benoy et al. [106][a]	RT-PCR	148	Pre-treatment	28,30%	No	CK-19 mRNA, mammaglobin
Ntoulia et al. [107]	RT-PCR	101	Pre-chemotherapy	13.9%	RFS	Mammaglobin A
Wiedswang et al. [108]	ICC	341	Pre-chemotherapy	10%	RFS and OS	AE1 and AE3
Wong et al. [109][a]	ICC	131	During chemotherapy	42,50%	No	CK-8
Xenidis et al. [110]	RT-PCR	167	Pre-chemotherapy	21,60%	RFS and OS	CK-19 mRNA
Ignatiadis et al. [30]	RT-PCR	444	Pre-chemotherapy	40.8%	RFS and OS	CK-19 mRNA
Xenidis et al. [111]	RT-PCR	119	Post-chemotherapy	18,15%	RFS and OS	CK-19 mRNA
Ignatiadis et al. [112]	RT-PCR	175	Pre-chemotherapy	41,1%/8%/28.6%	see text	CK-19, mammaglobin A and HER2
Tkaczuk et al. [113][a]	ICC	105	Pre- and post-chemotherapy	30% and 56%—post-24 months	OS	Multi-CK
Daskalaki et al. [114]	RT-PCR	165	Pre- and post-chemotherapy	55.2%	OS	CK-19mRNA
Marques et al. [115]	RT-PCR	321	Pre- and post-chemotherapy	55.1%	No	Mammaglobin mRNA
Serrano et al. [116][a]	ICC	71	Pre- and post-chemotherapy	66%	PFS and OS	CK

Xenidis et al. [31]	RT-PCR	437	Pre- and post-chemotherapy	41%/32%, respectively	RFS and OS	CK-19 mRNA
Bidard et al. [117]	CellSearch	115	Pre- and post-chemotherapy	23%	RFS and OS	CK-8, 18, 19 and CD45
Chen et al. [118]	RT-PCR	50	Pre-chemotherapy	54%	RFS	CK-19, mammaglobin and CEA
Molloy et al. [119]	RT-PCR	82	Pre-chemotherapy	20%	RFS	CK19, p1B, EGP-2, PS2, mammaglobin and SBEM
Molloy et al. [120]	RT-PCR	733	Pre-treatment	7.9%	RFS and OS	CK19, p1B, EGP-2, PS2, mammaglobin and SBEM
Lucci et al. [121]	CellSearch	302	Pre-chemotherapy	24%	RFS and OS	CK-8, 18, 19 and CD45
Aktas et al. [122]	AdnaTest	68	Pre-chemotherapy	31%	No	AdnaTest BC, EMT and SC
Rack et al. [123]	CellSearch	2026	Pre- and post-chemotherapy	21,5%/22.1%	RFS and OS	CK-8, 18, 19 and CD45
Tryfonidis et al. [124]	RT-PCR	223	Pre- and post-chemotherapy	44.4%/40.3	RFS and OS	CK-19 mRNA
Hartkopf et al. [125]	AdnaTest/CellSearch	202/383	Pre-chemotherapy	9%/5%	RFS for CellSearch	CK-8, 18, 19, CD45 and AdnaTest BC
Janni et al. [126]	CellSearch	3173	Pre-chemotherapy	20.2%	RFS and OS	CK-8,18,19 and CD45
Kasimir-Bauer et al. [127]	AdnaTest	376	Pre-chemotherapy	22%	RFS	AdnaTest BC
Kasimir-Bauer et al. [128]	AdnaTest	135	Pre- and post-chemotherapy	24%/8%	No	AdnaTest BC, EMT and SC

aBoth early and metastatic, *OS* overall survival, *CK* cytokeratin, *RT-PCR* reverse transcription-polymerase chain reaction, *ICC* immunocytochemistry, *RFS* relapse-free survival, *PFS* progression-free survival, *OS* overall survival, *BC* breast cancer, *EMT* epithelial-mesenchymal transition, *SC* stem cell, *CEA* carcinoembryogenic antigen

Table 2.2 Studies on HER2 status discordance between primary tumour and CTCs

Author	Number of patients	Disease setting	Method of detection	Number of discordant cases
Meng et al. [88]	57	Early and advanced	ICC	8
Riethdorf et al. [142]	213 and 207	Early	CellSearch	8 and 3
Lang et al. [140]	92	Early	CellSearch	0
Fehm et al. [136]	67	Advanced	AdnaTest	8
Wülfing et al. [144]	42	Early	ICC	12
Ignatiadis et al. [32]	174	Preinvasive and early	CellSearch	5
Pestrin et al. [141]	66	Advanced	CellSearch	8
Flores et al. [137]	75	Advanced	CellSearch	10
Kallergi et al. [138]	24	Early	ICC	10
Wallwiener et al. [143]	107	Advanced	ICC	27
Krishnamurthy et al. [139]	95	Early and advanced	CEE	5
Apostolaki et al. [134]	214	Early	RT-PCR	40
Apostolaki et al. [135]	2016	Early	RT-PCR	47
Ignatiadis et al. [30]	185	Early	RT-PCR	28

suggest additional specific treatment. We have demonstrated that different CTC subpopulations have different prognosis by studying 175 early BC patients using a three-marker (mammoglobin, HER2 and CK19) reverse transcriptase polymerase chain reaction (RT-PCR) (Table 2.1) [112].

Multiple markers have been investigated in both BC and other tumours that have led to ongoing interventional trials. Protein markers that have been investigated include HER2 and PDL1 [31, 32, 112, 130]. RNA expression and DNA mutation detection in CTCs have been performed in advanced prostate cancer and BC [131, 132].

For CTC characterisation, HER2 attracted attention because of the availability of specific agents of proven clinical value [133]. In parallel, it was uncovered that in some cases of HER2-negative primary tumours, HER2+ CTCs were detectable [30, 32, 88, 134–143] (Table 2.2).

Interventional Studies

Hypothetically, since CTC detection is a surrogate marker for replicating tumour cells, the detection of remaining CTCs after a course of chemotherapy can be taken as signifying suboptimal efficacy in the adjuvant or metastatic settings, and thus be used to select patients that need more extensive or different treatment. In parallel the existence of HER2-discordant CTC subpopulations has raised interest in trastuzumab treatment for CTC-positive women with an HER2-negative primary. This hypothesis has been explored and is under exploration in various trials [145] (Table 2.2).

Bozionelou and colleagues led a pilot study on 30 patients with advanced BC and detectable CTCs/DTCs 1 month post-latest treatment. Patients received trastuzumab alone. Of 20 patients receiving weekly trastuzumab, after 4 weeks 75% of patients had no detectable CTCs/DTCs and stopped treatment. Of 10 patients receiving 3-weekly trastuzumab, 60% had no detectable CTCs/DTCs and stopped treatment [146].

A similar single-centre study was conducted on the adjuvant setting, where 75 patients with HER2-negative primary tumour and detectable CTCs were randomised between post-adjuvant trastuzumab for 6 cycles or regular follow-up. Interestingly 89% of patients had HER2 overexpression in detected cells. 75% of patients in the treatment arm were CTC negative after the end of treatment, compared to 17.9% after the same time period in the control arm. Treatment arm was also significantly superior to control in terms of relapse-free survival [147].

An ongoing multicentre trial, the "Treat CTC" (NCT01548677), aims to confirm and extend the above results using the CellSearch technology. This is a phase II that is currently randomising HER2-negative BC patients with detectable CTCs irrespective of HER2 status after surgery and (neo)adjuvant chemotherapy to either 6 cycles of trastuzumab or observation. The primary objective of this trial is the rate of CTC detection post-treatment. The rationale and the design of the Treat CTC trial including the results of the pilot phase have been recently published [148].

Naume et al. aimed to evaluate the clinical utility of bone marrow DTCs in a large adjuvant trial in BC patients. 1066 patients were submitted to bone marrow biopsy after completing standard adjuvant chemotherapy with 5-FU, epirubicin and cyclophosphamide (FEC). A total of 7.2% were positive and went on to receive 6 cycles of docetaxel. Among these, 20.8% had persistent DTCs in bone marrow biopsy following docetaxel. Post-docetaxel, DTC-negative patients had similar prognosis to the group who were negative after FEC only, suggesting the effectiveness of this strategy [149].

Conclusions

Though recent advances in CTC/DTC research have shed new light in this process of dissemination, many hypotheses remain to be further tested. At this point in time it has been suggested that at least in some patients the detection and characterisation of CTCs/DTCs may provide additional information to that provided by the primary tumour alone. Ongoing or future studies using CTCs or newer more sensitive tools such as circulating tumour DNA will explore the question of tailoring adjuvant treatment for women with early breast cancer based on the detection of minimal residual disease. These studies, if positive, may change clinical practice in the early setting from a "static" primary biopsy-centric model to a "dynamic" liquid biopsy-centric model.

References

1. Torre LA, Bray F, Siegel RL, Ferlay J, Lortet-Tieulent J, Jemal A (2015) Global cancer statistics, 2012. CA Cancer J Clin 65:87–108
2. Hanahan D, Weinberg RA (2011) Hallmarks of cancer: the next generation. Cell 144:646–674
3. Valastyan S, Weinberg RA (2011) Tumor metastasis: molecular insights and evolving paradigms. Cell 147:275–292
4. Vogelstein B, Papadopoulos N, Velculescu VE, Zhou S, Diaz LA, Kinzler KW (2013) Cancer genome landscapes. Science 339:1546–1558
5. Ignatiadis M, Reinholz M (2011) Minimal residual disease and circulating tumor cells in breast cancer. Breast Cancer Res 13:222
6. Ignatiadis M, Lee M, Jeffrey SS (2015) Circulating tumor cells and circulating tumor DNA: challenges and opportunities on the path to clinical utility. Clin Cancer Res 21:4786–4800
7. Pantel K, Speicher MR (2016) The biology of circulating tumor cells. Oncogene 35(10):1216–1224
8. Arnedos M, Vicier C, Loi S, Lefebvre C, Michiels S, Bonnefoi H, Andre F (2015) Precision medicine for metastatic breast cancer--limitations and solutions. Nat Rev Clin Oncol 12:693–704
9. Schlange T, Pantel K (2016) Potential of circulating tumor cells as blood-based biomarkers in cancer liquid biopsy. Pharmacogenomics 17:183–186
10. Ashworth TR (1869) A case of cancer in which cells similar to those in the tumours were seen in the blood after death. Australian Medical Journal 14:146–147
11. Aceto N, Bardia A, Miyamoto DT, Donaldson MC, Wittner BS, Spencer JA, Yu M, Pely A, Engstrom A, Zhu H et al (2014) Circulating tumor cell clusters are oligoclonal precursors of breast cancer metastasis. Cell 158:1110–1122
12. Aguirre-Ghiso JA (2007) Models, mechanisms and clinical evidence for cancer dormancy. Nat Rev Cancer 7:834–846
13. Bednarz-Knoll N, Alix-Panabières C, Pantel K (2012) Plasticity of disseminating cancer cells in patients with epithelial malignancies. Cancer Metastasis Rev 31:673–687
14. Sosa MS, Bragado P, Aguirre-Ghiso JA (2014) Mechanisms of disseminated cancer cell dormancy: an awakening field. Nat Rev Cancer 14:611–622
15. Gupta GP, Massagué J (2006) Cancer metastasis: building a framework. Cell 127:679–695
16. Fisher B (2008) Biological research in the evolution of cancer surgery: a personal perspective. Cancer Res 68:10007–10020
17. Halsted WS (1894) I. The results of operations for the cure of cancer of the breast performed at the Johns Hopkins Hospital from June, 1889, to January, 1894. Ann Surg 20:497–555
18. Klein CA (2009) Parallel progression of primary tumours and metastases. Nat Rev Cancer 9:302–312
19. Fidler IJ, Kripke ML (1977) Metastasis results from preexisting variant cells within a malignant tumor. Science 197:893–895
20. Coates AS, Winer EP, Goldhirsch A, Gelber RD, Gnant M, Piccart-Gebhart M, Thürlimann B, Senn H-J (2015) Tailoring therapies—improving the management of early breast cancer: St Gallen International Expert Consensus on the Primary Therapy of Early Breast Cancer 2015. Ann Oncol 26:1533–1546
21. Oeffinger KC, Fontham ETH, Etzioni R, Herzig A, Michaelson JS, Shih Y-CT, Walter LC, Church TR, Flowers CR, LaMonte SJ et al (2015) Breast cancer screening for women at average risk: 2015 guideline update from the American Cancer Society. JAMA 314:1599
22. Weinberg RA (2008) Leaving home early: reexamination of the canonical models of tumor progression. Cancer Cell 14:283–284
23. Hanrahan EO, Gonzalez-Angulo AM, Giordano SH, Rouzier R, Broglio KR, Hortobagyi GN, Valero V (2007) Overall survival and cause-specific mortality of patients with stage T1a,bN0M0 breast carcinoma. J Clin Oncol 25:4952–4960

24. Hüsemann Y, Geigl JB, Schubert F, Musiani P, Meyer M, Burghart E, Forni G, Eils R, Fehm T, Riethmüller G et al (2008) Systemic spread is an early step in breast cancer. Cancer Cell 13:58–68
25. Klein CA (2013) Selection and adaptation during metastatic cancer progression. Nature 501:365–372
26. Banys M, Hahn M, Gruber I, Krawczyk N, Wallwiener M, Hartkopf A, Taran F-A, Röhm C, Kurth R, Becker S et al (2014) Detection and clinical relevance of hematogenous tumor cell dissemination in patients with ductal carcinoma in situ. Breast Cancer Res Treat 144:531–538
27. Sänger N, Effenberger KE, Riethdorf S, Van Haasteren V, Gauwerky J, Wiegratz I, Strebhardt K, Kaufmann M, Pantel K (2011) Disseminated tumor cells in the bone marrow of patients with ductal carcinoma in situ. Int J Cancer 129:2522–2526
28. Banys M, Gruber I, Krawczyk N, Becker S, Kurth R, Wallwiener D, Jakubowska J, Hoffmann J, Rothmund R, Staebler A et al (2012a) Hematogenous and lymphatic tumor cell dissemination may be detected in patients diagnosed with ductal carcinoma in situ of the breast. Breast Cancer Res Treat 131:801–808
29. Braun S, Vogl FD, Naume B, Janni W, Osborne MP, Coombes RC, Schlimok G, Diel IJ, Gerber B, Gebauer G et al (2005) A pooled analysis of bone marrow micrometastasis in breast cancer. N Engl J Med 353:793–802
30. Ignatiadis M, Xenidis N, Perraki M, Apostolaki S, Politaki E, Kafousi M, Stathopoulos EN, Stathopoulou A, Lianidou E, Chlouverakis G et al (2007) Different prognostic value of cyto-keratin-19 mRNA positive circulating tumor cells according to estrogen receptor and HER2 status in early-stage breast cancer. J Clin Oncol 25:5194–5202
31. Xenidis N, Ignatiadis M, Apostolaki S, Perraki M, Kalbakis K, Agelaki S, Stathopoulos EN, Chlouverakis G, Lianidou E, Kakolyris S et al (2009) Cytokeratin-19 mRNA-positive circulating tumor cells after adjuvant chemotherapy in patients with early breast cancer. J Clin Oncol 27:2177–2184
32. Ignatiadis M, Rothé F, Chaboteaux C, Durbecq V, Rouas G, Criscitiello C, Metallo J, Kheddoumi N, Singhal SK, Michiels S et al (2011) HER2-positive circulating tumor cells in breast cancer. PLoS One 6:e15624
33. Podsypanina K, Du Y-CN, Jechlinger M, Beverly LJ, Hambardzumyan D, Varmus H (2008) Seeding and propagation of untransformed mouse mammary cells in the lung. Science 321:1841–1844
34. Weng D, Penzner JH, Song B, Koido S, Calderwood SK, Gong J (2012) Metastasis is an early event in mouse mammary carcinomas and is associated with cells bearing stem cell markers. Breast Cancer Res 14:R18
35. van 't Veer LJ, Dai H, van de Vijver MJ, He YD, Hart AAM, Mao M, Peterse HL, van der Kooy K, Marton MJ, Witteveen AT et al (2002) Gene expression profiling predicts clinical outcome of breast cancer. Nature 415:530–536
36. Comen E, Norton L (2012) Self-seeding in cancer. Recent Results Cancer Res 195:13–23
37. Comen E, Norton L, Massagué J (2011) Clinical implications of cancer self-seeding. Nat Rev Clin Oncol 8:369–377
38. Sleeman JP, Nazarenko I, Thiele W (2011) Do all roads lead to Rome? Routes to metastasis development Int J Cancer 128:2511–2526
39. Kim M-Y, Oskarsson T, Acharyya S, Nguyen DX, Zhang XH-F, Norton L, Massagué J (2009) Tumor self-seeding by circulating cancer cells. Cell 139:1315–1326
40. Zhang Y, Ma Q, Liu T, Ke S, Jiang K, Wen Y, Ma B, Zhou Y, Fan Q, Qiu X (2014) Tumor self-seeding by circulating tumor cells in nude mouse models of human osteosarcoma and a preliminary study of its mechanisms. J Cancer Res Clin Oncol 140:329–340
41. Zhang Y, Ma Q, Liu T, Guan G, Zhang K, Chen J, Jia N, Yan S, Chen G, Liu S et al (2016) Interleukin-6 suppression reduces tumour self-seeding by circulating tumour cells in a human osteosarcoma nude mouse model. Oncotarget 7:446–458
42. Hartkopf AD, Wallwiener M, Fehm TN, Hahn M, Walter CB, Gruber I, Brucker SY, Taran F-A (2015) Disseminated tumor cells from the bone marrow of patients with nonmetastatic primary breast cancer are predictive of locoregional relapse. Ann Oncol 26:1155–1160

43. van Zijl F, Krupitza G, Mikulits W (2011) Initial steps of metastasis: cell invasion and endothelial transmigration. Mutat Res 728:23–34
44. Bockhorn M, Jain RK, Munn LL (2007) Active versus passive mechanisms in metastasis: do cancer cells crawl into vessels, or are they pushed? Lancet Oncol 8:444–448
45. Bryant DM, Mostov KE (2008) From cells to organs: building polarized tissue. Nat Rev Mol Cell Biol 9:887–901
46. Barriere G, Fici P, Gallerani G, Fabbri F, Rigaud M (2015) Epithelial Mesenchymal Transition: a double-edged sword. Clin Transl Med 4:14
47. Moustakas A, Heldin C-H (2007) Signaling networks guiding epithelial-mesenchymal transitions during embryogenesis and cancer progression. Cancer Sci 98:1512–1520
48. Thiery JP, Sleeman JP (2006) Complex networks orchestrate epithelial-mesenchymal transitions. Nat Rev Mol Cell Biol 7:131–142
49. De Craene B, Berx G (2013) Regulatory networks defining EMT during cancer initiation and progression. Nat Rev Cancer 13:97–110
50. Reymond N, d'Água BB, Ridley AJ (2013) Crossing the endothelial barrier during metastasis. Nat Rev Cancer 13:858–870
51. García de Herreros A (2014) Epithelial to mesenchymal transition in tumor cells as consequence of phenotypic instability. Front Cell Dev Biol 2:71
52. Egeblad M, Werb Z (2002) New functions for the matrix metalloproteinases in cancer progression. Nat Rev Cancer 2:161–174
53. Radisky ES, Radisky DC (2010) Matrix metalloproteinase-induced epithelial-mesenchymal transition in breast cancer. J Mammary Gland Biol Neoplasia 15:201–212
54. Mathias RA, Gopal SK, Simpson RJ (2013) Contribution of cells undergoing epithelial–mesenchymal transition to the tumour microenvironment. J Proteome 78:545–557
55. Sanz-Moreno V, Gadea G, Ahn J, Paterson H, Marra P, Pinner S, Sahai E, Marshall CJ (2008) Rac activation and inactivation control plasticity of tumor cell movement. Cell 135:510–523
56. Sabeh F, Shimizu-Hirota R, Weiss SJ (2009) Protease-dependent versus -independent cancer cell invasion programs: three-dimensional amoeboid movement revisited. J Cell Biol 185:11–19
57. Jolly MK, Boareto M, Huang B, Jia D, Lu M, Ben-Jacob E, Onuchic JN, Levine H (2015) Implications of the hybrid epithelial/mesenchymal phenotype in metastasis. Front Oncol 5:155
58. Gorges TM, Tinhofer I, Drosch M, Röse L, Zollner TM, Krahn T, von Ahsen O (2012) Circulating tumour cells escape from EpCAM-based detection due to epithelial-to-mesenchymal transition. BMC Cancer 12:178
59. Krawczyk N, Meier-Stiegen F, Banys M, Neubauer H, Ruckhaeberle E, Fehm T (2014) Expression of stem cell and epithelial-mesenchymal transition markers in circulating tumor cells of breast cancer patients. Biomed Res Int 2014:415721
60. Wu S, Liu S, Liu Z, Huang J, Pu X, Li J, Yang D, Deng H, Yang N, Xu J (2015) Classification of circulating tumor cells by epithelial-mesenchymal transition markers. PLoS One 10: e0123976
61. Cierna Z, Mego M, Janega P, Karaba M, Minarik G, Benca J, Sedláčková T, Cingelova S, Gronesova P, Manasova D et al (2014) Matrix metalloproteinase 1 and circulating tumor cells in early breast cancer. BMC Cancer 14:472
62. Duda DG, Duyverman AMMJ, Kohno M, Snuderl M, Steller EJA, Fukumura D, Jain RK (2010) Malignant cells facilitate lung metastasis by bringing their own soil. Proc Natl Acad Sci 107:21677–21682
63. Molnar B, Ladanyi A, Tanko L, Sréter L, Tulassay Z (2001) Circulating tumor cell clusters in the peripheral blood of colorectal cancer patients. Clin Cancer Res 7:4080–4085
64. Gupta GP, Nguyen DX, Chiang AC, Bos PD, Kim JY, Nadal C, Gomis RR, Manova-Todorova K, Massagué J (2007) Mediators of vascular remodelling co-opted for sequential steps in lung metastasis. Nature 446:765–770
65. Chambers AF, Groom AC, MacDonald IC (2002) Dissemination and growth of cancer cells in metastatic sites. Nat Rev Cancer 2:563–572

66. Méhes G, Witt A, Kubista E, Ambros PF (2001) Circulating breast cancer cells are frequently apoptotic. Am J Pathol 159:17–20
67. Tarin D, Price JE, Kettlewell MG, Souter RG, Vass AC, Crossley B (1984) Mechanisms of human tumor metastasis studied in patients with peritoneovenous shunts. Cancer Res 44:3584–3592
68. Paoli P, Giannoni E, Chiarugi P (2013) Anoikis molecular pathways and its role in cancer progression. Biochim Biophys Acta 1833:3481–3498
69. Lu D, Kassab GS (2011) Role of shear stress and stretch in vascular mechanobiology. J R Soc Interface 8:1379–1385
70. Mitchell MJ, King MR (2013a) Computational and experimental models of cancer cell response to fluid shear stress. Front Oncol 3:44
71. Mitchell MJ, King MR (2013b) Fluid shear stress sensitizes cancer cells to receptor-mediated apoptosis via trimeric death receptors. New J Phys 15:015008
72. Allen JE, Krigsfeld G, Patel L, Mayes PA, Dicker DT, Wu GS, El-Deiry WS (2015) Identification of TRAIL-inducing compounds highlights small molecule ONC201/TIC10 as a unique anti-cancer agent that activates the TRAIL pathway. Mol Cancer 14:99
73. Steinert G, Scholch S, Niemietz T, Iwata N, Garcia SA, Behrens B, Voigt A, Kloor M, Benner A, Bork U et al (2014) Immune escape and survival mechanisms in circulating tumor cells of colorectal cancer. Cancer Res 74:1694–1704
74. Tarin, D., Thompson, E.W., and Newgreen, D.F. (2005). The fallacy of epithelial mesenchymal transition in neoplasia. Cancer Res 65, 5996–6000; discussion 6000–6001
75. Cho EH, Wendel M, Luttgen M, Yoshioka C, Marrinucci D, Lazar D, Schram E, Nieva J, Bazhenova L, Morgan A et al (2012) Characterization of circulating tumor cell aggregates identified in patients with epithelial tumors. Phys Biol 9:016001
76. Paoletti C, Li Y, Muniz MC, Kidwell KM, Aung K, Thomas DG, Brown ME, Abramson VG, Irvin WJ, Lin NU et al (2015) Significance of circulating tumor cells in metastatic triple-negative breast cancer patients within a randomized, Phase II Trial: TBCRC 019. Clin Cancer Res 21:2771–2779
77. Hou J-M, Krebs M, Ward T, Sloane R, Priest L, Hughes A, Clack G, Ranson M, Blackhall F, Dive C (2011) Circulating tumor cells as a window on metastasis biology in lung cancer. Am J Pathol 178:989–996
78. Holen I, Whitworth J, Nutter F, Evans A, Brown HK, Lefley DV, Barbaric I, Jones M, Ottewell PD (2012) Loss of plakoglobin promotes decreased cell-cell contact, increased invasion, and breast cancer cell dissemination in vivo. Breast Cancer Res 14:R86
79. Hou J-M, Krebs MG, Lancashire L, Sloane R, Backen A, Swain RK, Priest LJC, Greystoke A, Zhou C, Morris K et al (2012) Clinical significance and molecular characteristics of circulating tumor cells and circulating tumor microemboli in patients with small-cell lung cancer. J Clin Oncol 30:525–532
80. Karachaliou N, Pilotto S, Bria E, Rosell R (2015) Platelets and their role in cancer evolution and immune system. Transl Lung Cancer Res 4:713–720
81. Riethdorf S, Pantel K (2008) Disseminated tumor cells in bone marrow and circulating tumor cells in blood of breast cancer patients: current state of detection and characterization. Pathobiology 75:140–148
82. Hadfield G (1954) The dormant cancer cell. Br Med J 2:607–610
83. Banys M, Hartkopf AD, Krawczyk N, Kaiser T, Meier-Stiegen F, Fehm T, Neubauer H (2012b) Dormancy in breast cancer. Breast Cancer (Dove Med Press) 4:183–191
84. Yeh AC, Ramaswamy S (2015) Mechanisms of cancer cell dormancy-another hallmark of cancer? Cancer Res 75:5014–5022
85. Naumov GN, Townson JL, MacDonald IC, Wilson SM, Bramwell VHC, Groom AC, Chambers AF (2003) Ineffectiveness of doxorubicin treatment on solitary dormant mammary carcinoma cells or late-developing metastases. Breast Cancer Res Treat 82:199–206
86. Zhang XH-F, Giuliano M, Trivedi MV, Schiff R, Osborne CK (2013) Metastasis dormancy in estrogen receptor-positive breast cancer. Clin Cancer Res 19:6389–6397

87. Rogers MS, Novak K, Zurakowski D, Cryan LM, Blois A, Lifshits E, Bø TH, Oyan AM, Bender ER, Lampa M et al (2014) Spontaneous reversion of the angiogenic phenotype to a nonangiogenic and dormant state in human tumors. Mol Cancer Res 12:754–764

88. Meng S, Tripathy D, Frenkel EP, Shete S, Naftalis EZ, Huth JF, Beitsch PD, Leitch M, Hoover S, Euhus D et al (2004) Circulating tumor cells in patients with breast cancer dormancy. Clin Cancer Res 10:8152–8162

89. Shiozawa Y, Nie B, Pienta KJ, Morgan TM, Taichman RS (2013) Cancer stem cells and their role in metastasis. Pharmacol Ther 138:285–293

90. Mitra A, Mishra L, Li S (2015) EMT, CTCs and CSCs in tumor relapse and drug-resistance. Oncotarget 6:10697–10711

91. Aktas B, Tewes M, Fehm T, Hauch S, Kimmig R, Kasimir-Bauer S (2009) Stem cell and epithelial-mesenchymal transition markers are frequently overexpressed in circulating tumor cells of metastatic breast cancer patients. Breast Cancer Res 11:R46

92. Giordano A, Gao H, Anfossi S, Cohen E, Mego M, Lee B-N, Tin S, De Laurentiis M, Parker CA, Alvarez RH et al (2012) Epithelial-mesenchymal transition and stem cell markers in patients with HER2-positive metastatic breast cancer. Mol Cancer Ther 11:2526–2534

93. Mani SA, Guo W, Liao M-J, Eaton EN, Ayyanan A, Zhou AY, Brooks M, Reinhard F, Zhang CC, Shipitsin M et al (2008) The epithelial-mesenchymal transition generates cells with properties of stem cells. Cell 133:704–715

94. Reuben JM, Lee B-N, Gao H, Cohen EN, Mego M, Giordano A, Wang X, Lodhi A, Krishnamurthy S, Hortobagyi GN et al (2011) Primary breast cancer patients with high risk clinicopathologic features have high percentages of bone marrow epithelial cells with ALDH activity and CD44+CD24lo cancer stem cell phenotype. Eur J Cancer 47:1527–1536

95. Kasimir-Bauer S, Hoffmann O, Wallwiener D, Kimmig R, Fehm T (2012) Expression of stem cell and epithelial-mesenchymal transition markers in primary breast cancer patients with circulating tumor cells. Breast Cancer Res 14:R15

96. Raimondi C, Gradilone A, Naso G, Vincenzi B, Petracca A, Nicolazzo C, Palazzo A, Saltarelli R, Spremberg F, Cortesi E et al (2011) Epithelial-mesenchymal transition and stemness features in circulating tumor cells from breast cancer patients. Breast Cancer Res Treat 130:449–455

97. Giordano A, Gao H, Cohen EN, Anfossi S, Khoury J, Hess K, Krishnamurthy S, Tin S, Cristofanilli M, Hortobagyi GN et al (2013) Clinical relevance of cancer stem cells in bone marrow of early breast cancer patients. Ann Oncol 24:2515–2521

98. Alix-Panabieres C, Pantel K (2016) Clinical applications of circulating tumor cells and circulating tumor DNA as liquid biopsy. Cancer Discov 6:479–491

99. Alix-Panabières C, Pantel K (2014) Challenges in circulating tumour cell research. Nat Rev Cancer 14:623–631

100. Stathopoulos EN, Sanidas E, Kafousi M, Mavroudis D, Askoxylakis J, Bozionelou V, Perraki M, Tsiftsis D, Georgoulias V (2005) Detection of CK-19 mRNA-positive cells in the peripheral blood of breast cancer patients with histologically and immunohistochemically negative axillary lymph nodes. Ann Oncol 16:240–246

101. Gaforio J-J, Serrano M-J, Sanchez-Rovira P, Sirvent A, Delgado-Rodriguez M, Campos M, de la Torre N, Algarra I, Dueñas R, Lozano A (2003) Detection of breast cancer cells in the peripheral blood is positively correlated with estrogen-receptor status and predicts for poor prognosis. Int J Cancer 107:984–990

102. Xenidis N, Vlachonikolis I, Mavroudis D, Perraki M, Stathopoulou A, Malamos N, Kouroussis C, Kakolyris S, Apostolaki S, Vardakis N et al (2003) Peripheral blood circulating cytokeratin-19 mRNA-positive cells after the completion of adjuvant chemotherapy in patients with operable breast cancer. Ann Oncol 14:849–855

103. Giatromanolaki A, Koukourakis MI, Kakolyris S, Mavroudis D, Kouroussis C, Mavroudi C, Perraki M, Sivridis E, Georgoulias V (2004) Assessment of highly angiogenic and disseminated in the peripheral blood disease in breast cancer patients predicts for resistance to adjuvant chemotherapy and early relapse. Int J Cancer 108:620–627

104. Pierga J-Y, Bonneton C, Vincent-Salomon A, de Cremoux P, Nos C, Blin N, Pouillart P, Thiery J-P, Magdelénat H (2004) Clinical significance of immunocytochemical detection of tumor cells using digital microscopy in peripheral blood and bone marrow of breast cancer patients. Clin Cancer Res 10:1392–1400

105. Masuda T-A, Kataoka A, Ohno S, Murakami S, Mimori K, Utsunomiya T, Inoue H, Tsutsui S, Kinoshita J, Masuda N et al (2005) Detection of occult cancer cells in peripheral blood and bone marrow by quantitative RT-PCR assay for cytokeratin-7 in breast cancer patients. Int J Oncol 26:721–730

106. Benoy IH, Elst H, Philips M, Wuyts H, Van Dam P, Scharpé S, Van Marck E, Vermeulen PB, Dirix LY (2006) Real-time RT-PCR detection of disseminated tumour cells in bone marrow has superior prognostic significance in comparison with circulating tumour cells in patients with breast cancer. Br J Cancer 94:672–680

107. Ntoulia M, Stathopoulou A, Ignatiadis M, Malamos N, Mavroudis D, Georgoulias V, Lianidou ES (2006) Detection of Mammaglobin A-mRNA-positive circulating tumor cells in peripheral blood of patients with operable breast cancer with nested RT-PCR. Clin Biochem 39:879–887

108. Wiedswang G, Borgen E, Schirmer C, Kåresen R, Kvalheim G, Nesland JM, Naume B (2006) Comparison of the clinical significance of occult tumor cells in blood and bone marrow in breast cancer. Int J Cancer 118:2013–2019

109. Wong NS, Kahn HJ, Zhang L, Oldfield S, Yang L-Y, Marks A, Trudeau ME (2006) Prognostic significance of circulating tumour cells enumerated after filtration enrichment in early and metastatic breast cancer patients. Breast Cancer Res Treat 99:63–69

110. Xenidis N, Perraki M, Kafousi M, Apostolaki S, Bolonaki I, Stathopoulou A, Kalbakis K, Androulakis N, Kouroussis C, Pallis T et al (2006) Predictive and prognostic value of peripheral blood cytokeratin-19 mRNA-positive cells detected by real-time polymerase chain reaction in node-negative breast cancer patients. J Clin Oncol Off J Am Soc Clin Oncol 24:3756–3762

111. Xenidis N, Markos V, Apostolaki S, Perraki M, Pallis A, Sfakiotaki G, Papadatos-Pastos D, Kalmanti L, Kafousi M, Stathopoulos E et al (2007) Clinical relevance of circulating CK-19 mRNA-positive cells detected during the adjuvant tamoxifen treatment in patients with early breast cancer. Ann Oncol 18:1623–1631

112. Ignatiadis M, Kallergi G, Ntoulia M, Perraki M, Apostolaki S, Kafousi M, Chlouverakis G, Stathopoulos E, Lianidou E, Georgoulias V et al (2008) Prognostic value of the molecular detection of circulating tumor cells using a multimarker reverse transcription-PCR assay for cytokeratin 19, mammaglobin A, and HER2 in early breast cancer. Clin Cancer Res 14:2593–2600

113. Tkaczuk KHR, Goloubeva O, Tait NS, Feldman F, Tan M, Lum Z-P, Lesko SA, Van Echo DA, Ts'o POP (2008) The significance of circulating epithelial cells in Breast Cancer patients by a novel negative selection method. Breast Cancer Res Treat 111:355–364

114. Daskalaki A, Agelaki S, Perraki M, Apostolaki S, Xenidis N, Stathopoulos E, Kontopodis E, Hatzidaki D, Mavroudis D, Georgoulias V (2009) Detection of cytokeratin-19 mRNA-positive cells in the peripheral blood and bone marrow of patients with operable breast cancer. Br J Cancer 101:589–597

115. Marques AR, Teixeira E, Diamond J, Correia H, Santos S, Neto L, Ribeiro M, Miranda A, Passos-Coelho JL (2009) Detection of human mammaglobin mRNA in serial peripheral blood samples from patients with non-metastatic breast cancer is not predictive of disease recurrence. Breast Cancer Res Treat 114:223–232

116. Serrano MJ, Sánchez-Rovira P, Delgado-Rodriguez M, Gaforio JJ (2009) Detection of circulating tumor cells in the context of treatment: prognostic value in breast cancer. Cancer Biol Ther 8:671–675

117. Bidard F-C, Mathiot C, Delaloge S, Brain E, Giachetti S, de Cremoux P, Marty M, Pierga J-Y (2010) Single circulating tumor cell detection and overall survival in nonmetastatic breast cancer. Ann Oncol 21:729–733

118. Chen Y, Zou TN, Wu ZP, Zhou YC, Gu YL, Liu X, Jin CG, Wang XC (2010) Detection of cytokeratin 19, human mammaglobin, and carcinoembryonic antigen-positive circulating tumor cells by three-marker reverse transcription-PCR assay and its relation to clinical outcome in early breast cancer. Int J Biol Markers 25:59–68

119. Molloy TJ, Bosma AJ, Baumbusch LO, Synnestvedt M, Borgen E, Russnes HG, Schlichting E, van 't Veer LJ, Naume B (2011a) The prognostic significance of tumour cell detection in the peripheral blood versus the bone marrow in 733 early-stage breast cancer patients. Breast Cancer Res 13:R61

120. Molloy TJ, Devriese LA, Helgason HH, Bosma AJ, Hauptmann M, Voest EE, Schellens JHM, van 't Veer LJ (2011b) A multimarker QPCR-based platform for the detection of circulating tumour cells in patients with early-stage breast cancer. Br J Cancer 104:1913–1919

121. Lucci A, Hall CS, Lodhi AK, Bhattacharyya A, Anderson AE, Xiao L, Bedrosian I, Kuerer HM, Krishnamurthy S (2012) Circulating tumour cells in non-metastatic breast cancer: a prospective study. Lancet Oncol 13:688–695

122. Aktas B, Bankfalvi A, Heubner M, Kimmig R, Kasimir-Bauer S (2013) Evaluation and correlation of risk recurrence in early breast cancer assessed by Oncotype DX(®), clinicopathological markers and tumor cell dissemination in the blood and bone marrow. Mol Clin Oncol 1:1049–1054

123. Rack B, Schindlbeck C, Jückstock J, Andergassen U, Hepp P, Zwingers T, Friedl TWP, Lorenz R, Tesch H, Fasching PA et al (2014) Circulating tumor cells predict survival in early average-to-high risk breast cancer patients. J Natl Cancer Inst 106

124. Tryfonidis K, Kafousi M, Perraki M, Apostolaki S, Agelaki S, Georgoulias V, Stathopoulos E, Mavroudis D (2014) Detection of circulating cytokeratin-19 mRNA-positive cells in the blood and the mitotic index of the primary tumor have independent prognostic value in early breast cancer. Clin Breast Cancer 14:442–450

125. Hartkopf AD, Wallwiener M, Hahn M, Fehm TN, Brucker SY, Taran F-A (2016) Simultaneous detection of disseminated and circulating tumor cells in primary breast cancer patients. Cancer Res Treat 48:115–124

126. Janni WJ, Rack B, Terstappen LWMM, Pierga J-Y, Taran F-A, Fehm T, Hall C, de Groot MR, Bidard F-C, Friedl TWP et al (2016) Pooled analysis of the prognostic relevance of circulating tumor cells in primary breast cancer. Clin Cancer Res 22:2583–2593

127. Kasimir-Bauer S, Bittner A-K, König L, Reiter K, Keller T, Kimmig R, Hoffmann O (2016a) Does primary neoadjuvant systemic therapy eradicate minimal residual disease? Analysis of disseminated and circulating tumor cells before and after therapy. Breast Cancer Res 18:20

128. Kasimir-Bauer S, Reiter K, Aktas B, Bittner A-K, Weber S, Keller T, Kimmig R, Hoffmann O (2016b) Different prognostic value of circulating and disseminated tumor cells in primary breast cancer: influence of bisphosphonate intake? Sci Rep 6:26355

129. Zhang L, Riethdorf S, Wu G, Wang T, Yang K, Peng G, Liu J, Pantel K (2012) Meta-analysis of the prognostic value of circulating tumor cells in breast cancer. Clin Cancer Res 18:5701–5710

130. Mazel M, Jacot W, Pantel K, Bartkowiak K, Topart D, Cayrefourcq L, Rossille D, Maudelonde T, Fest T, Alix-Panabières C (2015) Frequent expression of PD-L1 on circulating breast cancer cells. Mol Oncol 9:1773–1782

131. Antonarakis ES, Lu C, Wang H, Luber B, Nakazawa M, Roeser JC, Chen Y, Mohammad TA, Chen Y, Fedor HL et al (2014) AR-V7 and resistance to enzalutamide and abiraterone in prostate cancer. N Engl J Med 371:1028–1038

132. Schneck H, Blassl C, Meier-Stiegen F, Neves RP, Janni W, Fehm T, Neubauer H (2013) Analysing the mutational status of PIK3CA in circulating tumor cells from metastatic breast cancer patients. Mol Oncol 7:976–986

133. Piccart-Gebhart MJ, Procter M, Leyland-Jones B, Goldhirsch A, Untch M, Smith I, Gianni L, Baselga J, Bell R, Jackisch C et al (2005) Trastuzumab after adjuvant chemotherapy in HER2-positive breast cancer. N Engl J Med 353:1659–1672

134. Apostolaki S, Perraki M, Pallis A, Bozionelou V, Agelaki S, Kanellou P, Kotsakis A, Politaki E, Kalbakis K, Kalykaki A et al (2007) Circulating HER2 mRNA-positive cells in the peripheral blood of patients with stage I and II breast cancer after the administration of adjuvant chemotherapy: evaluation of their clinical relevance. Ann Oncol 18:851–858

135. Apostolaki S, Perraki M, Kallergi G, Kafousi M, Papadopoulos S, Kotsakis A, Pallis A, Xenidis N, Kalmanti L, Kalbakis K et al (2009) Detection of occult HER2 mRNA-positive tumor cells in the peripheral blood of patients with operable breast cancer: evaluation of their prognostic relevance. Breast Cancer Res Treat 117:525–534

136. Fehm T, Becker S, Duerr-Stoerzer S, Sotlar K, Mueller V, Wallwiener D, Lane N, Solomayer E, Uhr J (2007) Determination of HER2 status using both serum HER2 levels and circulating tumor cells in patients with recurrent breast cancer whose primary tumor was HER2 negative or of unknown HER2 status. Breast Cancer Res 9:R74

137. Flores LM, Kindelberger DW, Ligon AH, Capelletti M, Fiorentino M, Loda M, Cibas ES, Jänne PA, Krop IE (2010) Improving the yield of circulating tumour cells facilitates molecular characterisation and recognition of discordant HER2 amplification in breast cancer. Br J Cancer 102:1495–1502

138. Kallergi G, Agelaki S, Papadaki MA, Nasias D, Matikas A, Mavroudis D, Georgoulias V (2015) Expression of truncated human epidermal growth factor receptor 2 on circulating tumor cells of breast cancer patients. Breast Cancer Res 17:113

139. Krishnamurthy S, Bischoff F, Ann Mayer J, Wong K, Pham T, Kuerer H, Lodhi A, Bhattacharyya A, Hall C, Lucci A (2013) Discordance in HER2 gene amplification in circulating and disseminated tumor cells in patients with operable breast cancer. Cancer Med 2:226–233

140. Lang JE, Mosalpuria K, Cristofanilli M, Krishnamurthy S, Reuben J, Singh B, Bedrosian I, Meric-Bernstam F, Lucci A (2009) HER2 status predicts the presence of circulating tumor cells in patients with operable breast cancer. Breast Cancer Res Treat 113:501–507

141. Pestrin M, Bessi S, Galardi F, Truglia M, Biggeri A, Biagioni C, Cappadona S, Biganzoli L, Giannini A, Di Leo A (2009) Correlation of HER2 status between primary tumors and corresponding circulating tumor cells in advanced breast cancer patients. Breast Cancer Res Treat 118:523–530

142. Riethdorf S, Müller V, Zhang L, Rau T, Loibl S, Komor M, Roller M, Huober J, Fehm T, Schrader I et al (2010) Detection and HER2 expression of circulating tumor cells: prospective monitoring in breast cancer patients treated in the neoadjuvant GeparQuattro trial. Clin Cancer Res 16:2634–2645

143. Wallwiener M, Hartkopf AD, Riethdorf S, Nees J, Sprick MR, Schönfisch B, Taran F-A, Heil J, Sohn C, Pantel K et al (2015) The impact of HER2 phenotype of circulating tumor cells in metastatic breast cancer: a retrospective study in 107 patients. BMC Cancer 15:403

144. Wülfing P, Borchard J, Buerger H, Heidl S, Zänker KS, Kiesel L, Brandt B (2006) HER2-positive circulating tumor cells indicate poor clinical outcome in stage I to III breast cancer patients. Clin Cancer Res 12:1715–1720

145. Bidard F-C, Fehm T, Ignatiadis M, Smerage JB, Alix-Panabières C, Janni W, Messina C, Paoletti C, Müller V, Hayes DF et al (2013) Clinical application of circulating tumor cells in breast cancer: overview of the current interventional trials. Cancer Metastasis Rev 32:179–188

146. Bozionellou V, Mavroudis D, Perraki M, Papadopoulos S, Apostolaki S, Stathopoulos E, Stathopoulou A, Lianidou E, Georgoulias V (2004) Trastuzumab administration can effectively target chemotherapy-resistant cytokeratin-19 messenger RNA-positive tumor cells in the peripheral blood and bone marrow of patients with breast cancer. Clin Cancer Res 10:8185–8194

147. Georgoulias V, Bozionelou V, Agelaki S, Perraki M, Apostolaki S, Kallergi G, Kalbakis K, Xyrafas A, Mavroudis D (2012) Trastuzumab decreases the incidence of clinical relapses in patients with early breast cancer presenting chemotherapy-resistant CK-19mRNA-positive circulating tumor cells: results of a randomized phase II study. Ann Oncol 23:1744–1750

148. Ignatiadis M, Rack B, Rothé F, Riethdorf S, Decraene C, Bonnefoi H, Dittrich C, Messina C, Beauvois M, Trapp E et al (2016) Liquid biopsy-based clinical research in early breast cancer: the EORTC 90091-10093 Treat CTC trial. Eur J Cancer 63:97–104
149. Naume B, Synnestvedt M, Falk RS, Wiedswang G, Weyde K, Risberg T, Kersten C, Mjaaland I, Vindi L, Sommer HH et al (2014) Clinical outcome with correlation to disseminated tumor cell (DTC) status after DTC-guided secondary adjuvant treatment with docetaxel in early breast cancer. J Clin Oncol 32:3848–3857

Chapter 3
Enumeration and Molecular Analysis of CTCs in Metastatic Disease: The Breast Cancer Model

Cleo Parisi and Evi Lianidou

Abstract Molecular characterization of CTCs holds considerable promise for the identification of therapeutic targets and resistance mechanisms and for real-time monitoring of the efficacy of systemic therapies in patients with metastatic breast cancer. A variety of state-of-the-art systems are available for CTC isolation, detection, and molecular characterization. Analysis of CTCs at the gene expression, DNA methylation, and DNA mutation level holds considerable promise for an individualized treatment approach for patients with metastatic breast cancer.

Keywords Liquid biopsy • Circulating tumor cells (CTCs) • Enumeration • Molecular characterization • Single-cell analysis • Metastatic breast cancer • Individualized treatment

Introduction

Breast cancer (BrCa) is the most frequently diagnosed cancer and the leading cause of cancer death among females worldwide, with an estimated 1.7 million cases and 521,900 deaths in 2012 [1]. BrCa alone accounts for 29% of all cancer cases and 15% of all cancer deaths among females. Excluding skin cancers, BrCa is the most common cancer diagnosed among women in the USA, accounting for about one in three cancers, while about one in eight women in the USA will be diagnosed with BrCa in her lifetime [2, 3]. Approximately 246,660 new cases of female BrCa, about 61,000 cases of carcinoma in situ, and 40,450 deaths are expected among US women in 2016. BrCa is the leading cause of cancer death in women aged 20–59 years, but is replaced by lung cancer in women aged 60 years or older in the USA [2].

Metastasis causes about 90% of cancer deaths; however it is still the most enigmatic process of cancer pathogenesis. Patients with metastatic BrCa are mainly

C. Parisi • E. Lianidou, PhD (✉)
Department of Chemistry, Laboratory of Analytical Chemistry,
Analysis of Circulating Tumor Cells (ACTC) Lab, University of Athens, Athens, Greece
e-mail: k_parisi@chem.uoa.gr; lianidou@chem.uoa.gr

© Springer International Publishing AG 2017
M. Cristofanilli (ed.), *Liquid Biopsies in Solid Tumors*, Cancer Drug Discovery and Development, DOI 10.1007/978-3-319-50956-3_3

treated with systemic therapies, which can include chemotherapy, targeted therapy, and hormonal therapy. Thus, there is an urgent need for biomarkers towards the evaluation of diagnosis, prognosis, and real-time personalized monitoring of the efficacy of systemic adjuvant therapy.

Circulating tumor cells (CTCs) are the tumor cells that escape from the primary tumor—or a tumor in a distant site—and circulate in the patients' peripheral blood, thus giving rise to the hematogenous metastatic process. The presence of CTCs was first described in 1869 by the Australian physician Thomas Ashworth who observed microscopically "cells identical with those of the cancer itself" in the blood of a man with metastatic cancer [4]. However, it was not until the last decades that CTCs could be reliably and efficiently isolated and detected thanks to multiple technological advances. The presence of CTCs is already confirmed in patients before the detection of the primary tumor, during the recurrence of a carcinoma or even in patients who already had a primary tumor resection [5]. CTCs as major players in "liquid biopsy" [6] can provide significant information for a better understanding of tumor biology and cell dissemination and can serve as a useful tool for the detection, monitoring, and characterization of micrometastatic disease [7].

Detection of CTCs among millions of nonmalignant cells in a patient's blood sample represents a unique technical and analytical challenge. It is estimated that ~10^6 tumor cells per gram of tumor tissue enter daily into the bloodstream [8] and 1 mL of blood contains ~1 CTC in 10^5–10^8 leukocytes and ~10^9 erythrocytes [5]. Because of this rarity CTC enrichment is usually necessary in order to increase the sensitivity of any downstream CTC detection method. On the other hand, preprocessing of peripheral blood prior to CTC capture, such as by centrifugation or lysis of erythrocytes, can cause a reduction in capture efficiency and result in loss of CTCs. The approaches for CTC enrichment comprise a large panel of technologies based on their different characteristics distinguishing them from the surrounding normal hematopoietic cells, including physical (e.g., size, deformability, density, electric charges) and biological properties (e.g., cell surface protein expression, viability) and a variety of filtration devices and microfluidics as well. CTCs can be detected through imaging systems at the protein level (through specific antibodies) or through nucleic acid-based approaches. CTC enumeration alone is not enough in most cases and the molecular characterization of CTCs is necessary to provide important information on their molecular and biological nature.

In this chapter we focus on the main systems and platforms used for CTC isolation and detection, and the clinical significance of their enumeration and molecular characterization in metastatic breast cancer.

Enrichment, Isolation, and Detection of CTCs

CTC enrichment and detection systems can be broadly categorized as (a) label dependent, using positive enrichment with cell surface markers such as the epithelial cell adhesion molecule (EpCAM), and (b) label independent, where the enrichment of CTCs is based on negative selection, size, or other biophysical properties (Fig. 3.1. and Fig. 3.2.).

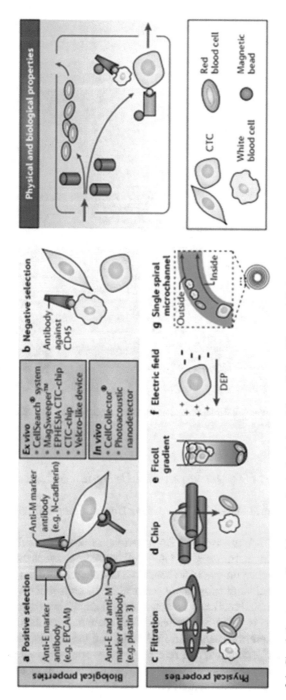

Fig. 3.1 Circulating tumor cell enrichment technologies (adapted from C. Panabières and K. Pantel, Nat Reviews Cancer, Perspective, 2014)

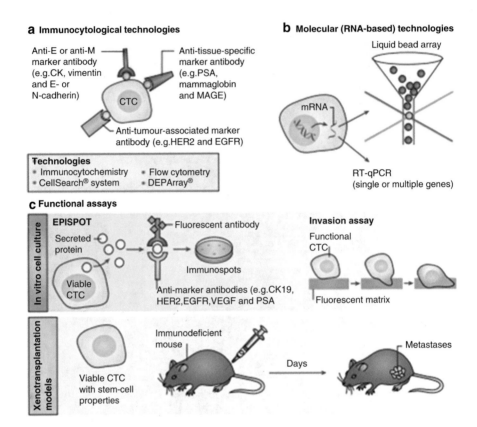

Fig. 3.2 Circulating tumor cell detection technologies (adapted from C. Panabières and K. Pantel, Nat Reviews Cancer, Perspective, 2014)

Label-Dependent CTC Isolation and Detection Systems

CTC Enrichment and Detection by Positive Immunomagnetic Selection

In this approach, CTCs are isolated from peripheral blood cells through specific antibodies which target tumor-associated cell surface antigens like EpCAM or MUC-1 and are attached on magnetic beads. CTC isolation is based on the application of a magnetic field and subsequent removal of the cells that do not carry these cancer-specific epithelial markers. The main advantage of this approach is the ease of use and the option to be fully automated. The main disadvantage is the fact that CTCs that do not express these specific epithelial antigens cannot be isolated.

The CellSearch® system. When referring to the term "CTC enumeration," the first technology that comes in mind is the CellSearch® system recently aquired by Memarini Silicon Biosystems which combines CTC isolation and detection in a semi-automated way. Although there is nowadays an ever-growing number of different platforms and devices of high sensitivity, CellSearch® is still the only FDA-approved system for CTC isolation and detection for metastatic breast [9], prostate [10, 11], and colorectal cancer [12]; thus it is established as the "gold standard" in the field and the majority of the emerging platforms compare their results to CellSearch® to validate their approaches. The CellSearch® system uses ferrofluid nanoparticles functionalized with an EpCAM antibody to allow magnetic separation of EpCAM-positive cells from solid blood components following centrifugation of 7.5 mL of blood. CTCs are then detected among the captured cells by a combination of immunocytochemistry and immunofluorescence to confirm the expression of cytokeratins (CK-8, CK-18, and CK-19) as epithelial specific markers, of DAPI as a nuclear stain, as well as the lack of CD-45 expression. Another main strength of this system is the possibility for further characterization of isolated CTCs by performing an additional analysis with a monoclonal antibody of interest in the fourth channel, such as in the recent detection of PD-L1 in CTCs of BrCa patients [13]. As a semi-automated platform for CTC detection, the variability among the readers in image interpretation represents a main concern in inter-laboratory studies. The international study which evaluated the inter-reader agreement in the classification of CellSearch® images as CTCs and interpretation of HER2 staining on them provided a high agreement for CTCs although it was reduced in nonmetastatic patients with low CTC counts suggesting the need for continuous training and independent image review [14].

AdnaTest® (Qiagen, Germany) is a series of commercially available assays that combine the immunomagnetic enrichment of CTCs and subsequent multiplex RT-PCR assays. This approach offers the possibility to simultaneously characterize cells for several additional markers. AdnaTest enriches CTCs through the use of magnetic beads, coated with a cocktail of Abs, such as EpCAM and MUC-1, specific to the type of cancer or EMT/stem cell. Following selection, captured CTCs are lysed and tested for expression patterns of various cancer-associated tumor markers (breast: GA733–2 (EpCAM), MUC-1, and HER2/prostate: PSMA, PSA, EGFR, and AR [15]/ovarian: GA733–2, MUC-1, CA125, and ERCC1/colon: GA733–2, CEA, and EGFR [16]/EMT/stem cell: PIK3Cα, AKT-2, TWIST, and ALDH1 [17, 18] and β-actin as a reference gene using multiplex RT-PCR). The test is not quantitative, and the detection of PCR transcripts is based on the Bioanalyzer electrophoresis approach. A sample is considered positive for the presence of CTCs if a PCR fragment of at least one tumor-associated transcript is clearly detected. Using the software package for the evaluation of the data on the Agilent 2100 Bioanalyzer, peaks with a concentration of >0.15 ng/μL are positive for the transcripts GA733–2, MUC-1, and HER2 in AdnaTest BreastCancer [19].

MagSweeper isolates CTCs with relatively high purity and is capable of processing whole blood without erythrocyte lysis or centrifugation. Antibody-coated magnetic beads are mixed with the blood sample to capture CTCs. A magnetic rod isolates captured CTCs by sweeping through wells containing the mixture of blood and beads, eliminating the unbound cells. The MagSweeper can process a blood sample at a rate of 9 mL/h, and it can be scaled up to process multiple samples in parallel through an automatically controlled array of magnetic rods [20].

Microfluidic Based Positive CTC Enrichment

There is a great variety of microfluidic devices and chips applied in the CTC isolation field. These devices are using micropost arrays or surfaces coated with specific antibodies against epithelial antigens, such as EpCAM. The **CTC-Chip** was the first micro-fluidic device based on this approach, isolating CTCs with a purity of 50%, and a low specificity, since a very high number of positive findings in healthy individuals was reported [21]. In an optimized version, the same group presented the **HB (herringbone)-chip** that was based on a passive mixing of peripheral blood cells through the generation of microvortices to significantly increase the number of interactions between targeted CTC population and the antibody-coated chip surface [22]. The **CTC-iChip** developed by the same group uses hydrodynamic size-based sorting, inertial focusing, and immunomagnetophoresis for CTC enrichment [23]. The **geometrically enhanced differential immunocapture (GEDI)** device also uses hydrodynamic chromatography for size-based cell separation and was first designed for prostate cancer CTCs [24].

In Vivo Positive Enrichment Technologies

The **CellCollector**™ (GILUPI GmbH, Germany) is a unique in vivo technology for CTC isolation overcoming the limitation of the small blood sample volumes used in the great majority of ex vivo approaches. It consists of a functionally structured medical nanowire (FSMW, Seldinger guidewire) which is placed intravenously in the patient for 30 min. In this way, 1.5 L of blood is able to pass the 2 cm functionalized area of the nanodetector with an anti-EpCAM antibody to trap CTCs as they flow by, thus enabling a high number of CTCs to be bound [25].

CTC Enrichment by Negative Selection (Label-Independent Techniques)

Negative selection technologies remove background cells by targeting antigens not expressed by CTCs, such as CD45. Thus, the antibody used in this process does not bias the subpopulation of isolated CTCs; however this approach for CTC enrichment usually yields cells of lower purity compared to positive enrichment systems. There is a number of immunomagnetic positive enrichment technologies that can be equally used for negative enrichment by changing the antibody (e.g., replacing anti-EpCAM with anti-CD45), with no need for further modifications to the device, such as the CTC-iChip [26].

CTC Enrichment Based on Biophysical Properties (Label-Independent Techniques)

Size- and/or Deformability-Based Enrichment of CTCs (Microfiltration Systems)

Size-based CTC enrichment technologies function on the principle that CTCs generally present a larger morphology than white blood cells [27]. Microfabrication methods have provided more sophisticated techniques for generating microfilters, e.g., lithography (optical, X-ray, colloidal), track-etching (polymer, silicon wafer, reactive ion), electrospinning, vapor-phase coating, and gas foaming [28]. Microfiltration systems allow rapid processing of blood for CTC enrichment but the overlap in size distributions between white blood cells and CTCs results in relatively low purity levels (<10%) while these systems are susceptible to clogging. Cell deformability may affect the performance of microfiltration technologies because cells may penetrate membrane pores unless stiffened by chemical fixation. Inertial focusing is also a size-based approach for viable CTC microfluidic enrichment making use of lift forces depending on channel dimensions and aspect ratio, flow rate, and particle diameter [26].

   ISET (isolation by size of epithelial tumor cells) system filters fixed samples through 8 mm pores in track-etched 0.6 cm diameter membranes in 10–12 wells able to process 1 mL volume. The ISET system maintains cell integrity allowing for CTC detection and cytological staining, cytopathological analysis, and further characterization [29]. ScreenCell® filters fixed or live samples through circular track-etched hydrophilic membranes with 7.5 mm or 6.5 mm pores, respectively. Depending on the filter used, there is the possibility for subsequent cytological studies (ScreenCell®Cyto), live cell culture (ScreenCell®CC), and molecular biology assays (ScreenCell®MB) [30]. Parsortix® (Angle) is a 3D microfiltration system using a disposable cassette to capture and then harvest CTCs. CTCs are caught on a step that crisscrosses the microscope slide-sized cassette. Captured cells can be fixed and stained in the cassette for identification and enumeration, or alternatively can be recovered for external staining and/or genetic analyses such as qPCR or sequencing [31].

Centrifugation

The term "density-based gradient centrifugation" refers to the use of buoyancy to separate different particles based on their relative densities. There is a variety of commercially available reagents used as an initial CTC enrichment step, such as Ficoll-Paque® (GE Healthcare Life Sciences, USA) and Lymphoprep™ (STEMCELL Technologies, Canada). OncoQuick® (Grenier Bio-One, Germany) is a combination of density-based gradient centrifugation and filtration by using a porous membrane on top of the separation media, which captures CTCs while allowing red and some white blood cells to pass through [32]. The RosetteSep™

CTC Enrichment Cocktail (STEMCELL Technologies, Canada) is a unique immunodensity approach that uses tetrameric antibody complexes to cross-link unwanted cells with erythrocytes. Using a standard density gradient medium (e.g., Ficoll-Paque® or Lymphoprep™) these cells sink to the bottom and the CTCs can be recovered from the plasma and density gradient medium interphase [33].

Dielectrophoresis (DEP)

DEP is based on the electrical properties of different cells, depending on their size, cell membrane, shape, density, and phenotype. The **DEPArray™** (Menarini Silicon Biosystems, Italy) platform is the only automated system for single-cell recovery and traps the cells in DEP cages generated by arrayed electrodes [34]. Like the CellSearch® system, the DEPArray™ platform has integrated a direct imaging approach for CTC detection using high-resolution fluorescence imaging. These two systems are frequently combined for bulk CTC isolation followed by single-cell isolation, respectively (described in detail in section "Single-Cell Analysis in Metastatic BrCa Patients").

Imaging Systems for CTC Analysis

There is also a number of imaging platforms which achieved to eliminate the CTC enrichment process thanks to the progress made in multiparameter fluorescence imaging. Examples of imaging platforms are the **FASTCell™** (SRI Biosciences, USA), a fiber-optic array scanning technology detecting CTCs through multiple tumor biomarkers [35], and the **CytoTrack™** (CytoTrack ApS, Denmark) system, which spins the special glass disc CytoDisc™ like a CD/DVD and scan 100 million cells/min on its surface through a laser [36]. A particular label-independent method for CTC detectio n is the **photoacoustic flow cytometry** (**PAFC**). In this system, a laser-based technology scans the veins through the skin as the blood flows; the cells present in the bloodstream absorb the laser radiation increasing their temperature leading to acoustic wave creation, detected by a nearby ultrasound device [37]. PAFC, like the CellCollector™, can detect CTCs in larger blood volumes in contrast to ex vivo approaches.

Functional Assays

Functional assays are based on traits of live cells for their isolation and/or detection.

The **EPISPOT** (**EPIthelial immunoSPOT**) technique allows the detection of viable clinically relevant CTCs enriched by leukocyte depletion, thus enabling the detection of EpCAM-positive and EpCAM-negative CTCs as well. The cells are cultured for a short time (48 h) on a nitrocellulose membrane coated with antibodies that capture the secreted/released/shed tumor-associated proteins that are subsequently detected by secondary antibodies labeled with fluorochromes. For BrCa, CK-19, HER-2, cathepsin D, and MUC-1 have been used as marker proteins [38, 39]. For prostate cancer, PSA has been used for CTC detection [40] and FGF2 as stem cell growth factor for further characterization [41]. For colorectal cancer, CK19 has been used for CTC detection [42]. By adding drugs in the EPISPOT assay, the number and intensity of the immunospots can be decreased or inhibited when tumor cells are sensitive to these drugs, demonstrating their efficiency during short-time CTC culture.

Another approach, for the in vivo study of CTCs, is based on **patient-derived xenografts** that can be used as tractable systems for therapy testing and understanding drug resistance mechanisms [43]. Applying this approach to CTCs has led to the development of unique in vivo models for several cancer types [44–46].

An alternative approach for CTC isolation is the process of **leukapheresis** which is based on the collection of mononuclear cells with a density of 1.055–1.08 g/mL from peripheral blood via continuous centrifugation. CTCs as epithelial cells have a similar density; thus they can be harvested along with the mononuclear cells during this procedure. The CTCs can subsequently be elutriated for ex vivo CTC analyses using flow cytometry and real-time PCR for molecular characterization [47].

Many more platforms and devices for CTC isolation and detection are excellently reviewed in recent publications [26, 48].

Clinical Significance of CTC Enumeration in Metastatic BrCa

The significant clinical validity of CTC count has been shown undoubtedly by Cristofanilli et al. in 2004, leading the FDA to clear the CellSearch® system for CTC detection in metastatic BrCa. In this seminal paper, CTC count was assessed for 177 patients starting a new line of treatment, at baseline and after few weeks of treatment [9]. The cutoff value to distinguish patients with short vs. long PFS was investigated and set up at ≥5 CTCs/7.5 mL of blood on the basis of a training cohort and was confirmed in a validation cohort. Considering the threshold of ≥5 or <5 CTCs at baseline and after 1 cycle of treatment as well, four different PFS profiles could be distinguished. As expected, the worse prognosis was observed in patients with ≥5 CTCs/7.5 mL at both time points. However, patients with high CTC levels at baseline but with a low CTC count after 1 cycle of therapy had a much better prognosis, almost similar to that of patients with low CTC count at baseline. The same cutoff value was used for follow-up CTC counts during treatment. High CTC counts during any time of the treatment have shown a poor prognosis for metastatic BrCa patients [49].

A recent pooled analysis of 1.944 individual patient data demonstrated for the first time the superiority of CTC count over serum tumor markers (CEA, CA15–3). CTC count is associated with performance status, number of metastatic sites, elevated LDH, and elevated serum tumor markers while ≥ 1 CTC could be detected in about 70% of stage IV BrCa patients. In this study, CTC levels were reported as a dynamic prognostic marker of PFS and OS [50].

The use of CTC enumeration by clinicians was recently seriously affected by the negative results of the Southwest Oncology Group (SWOG) S0500 clinical trial. The value of CTC enumeration for treatment decision making was prospectively tested in metastatic BrCa patients whose CTC level stayed >5/7.5 mL of blood after the first cycle of the first line of chemotherapy. The patients were eventually randomized to an early switch to the second line of chemotherapy, supposing that this switch would greatly improve their OS compared to the standard imaging-based management. However, this hypothesis was not proved correct as no survival difference was observed between the two arms [51]. However, this apparent "failure" of CTC count to benefit metastatic BrCa patients is not due to CTCs per se but it represents a result of the absence of a better treatment for these patients [48].

CTC-directed therapies are also an attractive approach that could be implemented in the clinical practice. For example, it is well known that HER2-positive CTCs can be detected in patients with HER2-negative primary tumors [52, 53]. In this context, a multicenter phase II clinical trial in metastatic BrCa patients has investigated the possible benefit of lapatinib monotherapy, but almost none of the screened patients presented a significant response [54]. Lapatinib administration in metastatic BrCa patients with therapy-resistant HER2-positive CTCs resulted in a reduction in HER2-positive CTC counts independently of the primary tumor status, but no clinical objective response was observed [55]. Similar results are reported in another phase II clinical trial investigating whether lapatinib as a single-agent treatment could have an impact in metastatic BrCa patients with HER2-negative primary tumors and EGFR-positive CTCs. In this case too, although the number of EGFR-positive CTCs was lower after the treatment, there was no clinical effect for the patients [56]. In contrast, the administration of gefitinib in metastatic BrCa patients with EGFR-positive CTCs resulted in lower number of CTCs regardless of their EGFR status while two patients had prolonged PFS and one showed clinical objective response [57].

Whether an early change in chemotherapy regimen based on CTC levels in the third line or later setting would impact prognostic outcome is currently being investigated in the CirCe01 trial while another French study, the STIC CTC METABREAST, investigates the clinical utility of the prognostic value of baseline CTC count. In this trial, the choice of the first line of treatment (hormono- or chemotherapy) for relapsing hormone-positive BrCa is determined either by the clinician or the baseline CTC enumeration [58, 59].

In Table 3.1 the clinical studies based on the enumeration of CTCs in metastatic BrCa are presented.

Table 3.1 CTC enumeration studies in metastatic BrCa patients (based on [7, 110, 111])

Author	Method	Markers	Patients number	Positivity rate (%)	Prognostic significance	
					PFS	OS
Cristofanilli et al. [9]	CellSearch®		177	49	Yes	Yes
Cristofanilli et al. [112]	CellSearch®		83	52	Yes	Yes
De Giorgi et al. [113]	CellSearch®		195	47	Yes	Yes
Budd et al. [114]	CellSearch®		138	25	No	Yes
Giordano et al. [115]	CellSearch®		517	40	Yes	Yes
Wallwiener et al. [116]	CellSearch®		486	42	Yes	Yes
Pierga et al. [117]	CellSearch®		267	44	Yes	Yes
Giuliano et al. [118]	CellSearch®		235	40	Yes	Yes
Hayes et al. [49]	CellSearch®		177	54	Yes	Yes
Nakamura et al. [119]	CellSearch®		107	37	Yes	No
Nole et al. [120]	CellSearch®		80	61	Yes	No
Liu et al. [121]	CellSearch®		74	–	Yes	No
Müller et al. [105]	CellSearch®		254	50	No	Yes
Munzone et al. [122]	CellSearch®	HER2	45	18	Yes	NA
Fehm et al. [94]	CellSearch®	HER2	254	50	NA	NA
Punnoose et al. [53]	CellSearch®, IF, FISH	HER2	38	76	NA	NA
Pestrin et al. [52]	CellSearch®, IF, FISH	HER2	52	70	NA	NA

Molecular Characterization of CTCs in Metastatic BrCa: Clinical Significance

There is no doubt that different methodologies detect different cell populations due to the great heterogeneity present in CTCs [60, 61]. Moreover, enrichment and detection are mostly based on epithelial markers, such as the EpCAM and specific cytokeratins, resulting in lack of detection of those CTCs that have undergone EMT, and lost—partially or totally—their epithelial characteristics, by conventional methods [18, 62]. Breast CTCs may also express cytokeratins in complex patterns so that clinically important subsets may be missed when individual anti-CK antibodies are used for their isolation [63]. Therefore, CTC enumeration alone is not enough in most cases and the molecular characterization of CTCs is necessary to provide important information on the molecular and biological nature of these cells.

Molecular characterization of CTCs is of great importance for the confirmation of their malignant origin, the real-time monitoring of immunophenotypic changes with tumor progression, and stratification of cancer patients in order to receive personalized treatment through diagnostically and therapeutically relevant targets. Individual tailored treatments based on the molecular characterization of CTCs could not only improve their efficacy [64] but monitor markers of resistance to targeted therapies [65] and predict early response to therapy as well [19]. The molecular characterization of CTCs is highly promising especially in combination with NGS technologies that will enable the elucidation of molecular pathways in CTCs, and will probably lead to the design of novel molecular therapies specifically targeting CTCs. Even if this is still far from being considered for application in a routine clinical setting, it holds great promise for the future management of cancer patients [7].

The molecular characterization of CTCs as a bulk or single CTCs is feasible at the following levels: (a) RNA level for gene expression, (b) DNA level for genetic alterations, and (c) epigenetic level for DNA methylation studies. In Table 3.2 a number of studies for the molecular characterization of CTCs in metastatic BrCa are presented.

Table 3.2 Molecular characterization of CTCs in metastatic BrCa patients (based on [7, 111, 123])

Author	Methods	Markers	Prognostic significance	
			PFS	OS
Müller et al. [105]	AdnaTest BreastCancer		No	No
Tewes et al. [19]	AdnaTest BreastCancer		No	Yes
Reinholz et al. [124]	RT-PCR	CK19 / hMAM	No	Yes
Benoy et al. [125]	RT-PCR	CK19	No	No
Pierga et al. [126]	RT-PCR	CK19, MUC-1	NA	Yes
Bidard et al. [127]	ICC	CKs	No	Yes
Li et al. [128]	IHC, FISH	AR, ER, Ki67, HER2	No	NA
Sieuwerts et al. [129]	CellSearch®, RT-PCR	55 mRNAs and 10 miRNAs	NA	NA
Meng et al. [130]	FISH	uPAR, HER2	NA	NA
Kallergi et al. [131]	IF	CK, TWIST, VIM	NA	NA
Aktas et al. [17]	AdnaTest BreastCancer and EMT-1/StemCell		NA	NA
Theodoropoulos et al. [132]	IF	CD44/CD24, ALDH1	NA	NA
Kallergi et al. [133]	Confocal laser scanning microscopy, RT-PCR	VEGF, VEGF-2, HIF-1, pFAK	NA	NA

Gene Expression Studies in CTCs from Metastatic BrCa Patients

RT-PCR and RT-qPCR have been widely used to detect the presence of CTCs and also for their specific molecular characterization. The target transcripts used for CTC detection are predominantly of either epithelial- or tissue-specific origin and therefore presumably not transcribed by contaminating leukocytes. The ability to multiplex this approach and examine multiple genes at once within a given reaction mixture from a very small initial sample volume is a significant advantage that this technique offers after a careful and detailed in silico design [66, 67]. Multiplexed assays are widely used for molecular characterization of CTCs [19, 61, 68, 69]. A multiplex RT-qPCR assay for the simultaneous detection of *CK19, HER2, MAGEA3*, and *PBGD* transcripts has been developed for CTC molecular characterization in breast cancer patients [61].

Another approach using multiplex PCR is the liquid bead array (Luminex® System, Luminex® Corporation, USA) that is automated and often present in clinical laboratories for a variety of applications [70]. A highly sensitive and specific assay based on a multiplex PCR coupled to a liquid bead array has been developed and validated for the molecular characterization of BrCa CTCs [71]. The assay detects simultaneously the expression of *CK19, HER2, hMAM, MAGEA3, TWIST*, and *PBGD* as a reference gene. This assay has been expanded for the detection of eight more genes, involving targets for stemness and EMT [72].

The clinical significance of CTCs in metastatic BrCa patients has been shown not only by CTC enumeration but by using RT-PCR as well. Before the initiation of front-line treatment in patients with metastatic BrCa, the median PFS and OS were significantly shorter when CK-19 mRNA-positive CTCs were detected compared with patients that were negative for CK-19 mRNA [73]. Moreover, the detection of viable CTCs that secrete CK19 correlates with OS using the EPISPOT assay [74].

Mutation Detection Studies in CTCs from Metastatic BrCa Patients

DNA mutations are commonly studied in ctDNA, as a direct source of malignant origin, and in single tumor cells (as described in section "Single-Cell Analysis in Metastatic BrCa Patients"), reflecting a mutational heterogeneity between the cells shed from the primary tumor and the primary tumor itself. A couple of studies report alterations in DNA isolated from bulk CTCs and more specifically for *PIK3CA*. *PIK3CA* mutations are recognized as part of the resistance mechanism in anti-HER2 treatment in HER2-positive BrCa patients.

Schneck et al. using the CellSearch® system isolated CTCs from metastatic BrCa patients in the context of a translational spin-off study based on the DETECT III trial [75]. The SnaPshot assay was used to detect *PIK3CA* mutations in exons 9 and 20, after DNA extraction and WGA, revealing a mutational heterogeneity between different patients and in the same patient as well. Recently, a highly sensitive and specific methodology for the detection of *PIK3CA* hot-spot mutations in CTCs was developed that was based on the use of an allele-specific, asymmetric rapid PCR along with HRMA [76]. This study highlighted these mutations as a frequent event in early and metastatic BrCa patients as well, while in the latter, mutated CTCs were correlated with worse OS.

DNA Methylation Studies in CTCs from Metastatic BrCa Patients

The epigenetic state of CTCs has only started to be studied during the last decade and the number of these studies is so far very limited [81, 90]. This could be explained by the combined technical challenges of CTC isolation and DNA methylation analyses on extremely rare cells [77]. A series of three studies using MSP investigated for the first time the methylation status of three tumor-associated gene promoters in CTCs from patients with BrCa:

1. **Cystatin E/M** (encoded by ***CST6***), a cystatin of the type 2 (extracellular) family, is an endogenous cysteine cathepsin inhibitor which ensures protection of cells and tissues against the proteolytic activity of lysosomal peptidases [78]. *CST6* has been assigned to chromosome region 11q13, which is the site of **loss of heterozygosity** (**LOH**) in several types of cancer and is believed to harbor tumor-suppressor genes [79]. Hypermethylation of this region leads to under-expression of cystatin M in many cancers including BrCa [80]. It has been demonstrated that *CST6* is epigenetically silenced in CTCs of operable and metastatic BrCa patients [81].

2. **Breast cancer metastasis suppressor 1** (***BRMS1***) reduces the metastatic potential, but not the tumorigenicity, of human BrCa and melanoma cell lines. This gene encodes a predominantly nuclear protein involved in repressing transcription [82] and regulation of expression of multiple metastasis-associated miRNAs [83]. BRMS1 also inhibits NF-κB activity [84], EGFR expression, and downstream Akt signaling [85]. It has been demonstrated that *BRMS1* promoter is methylated in CTCs of BrCa patients [81, 86].

3. **SRY (sex-determining region Y)-box 17** (***SOX17***) encodes a member of the SOX family of transcription factors involved in embryogenesis, survival and differentiation of the definitive endoderm of early embryo, and determination of the cell fate [87]. The encoded protein is involved in the regulation of the canonical Wnt/β-catenin signaling pathway [88]. *SOX17* silencing occurs through pro-

moter methylation in many types of cancer including BrCa [89]. *SOX17* promoter was found hypermethylated in CTCs of operable and metastatic BrCa patients [90].

Very recently a liquid bead array assay combined with a multiplex MSP was developed for the evaluation of the methylation status of *CST6*, *BRMS1*, and *SOX17* promoters in CTCs [91].

Single-Cell Analysis in Metastatic BrCa Patients

The small number of isolated CTCs is the most important limitation for a successful molecular characterization; CTC numbers are even smaller in patients with lower tumor load such as in early-stage disease.

Single-cell gene expression analysis offers the opportunity to study tumor heterogeneity and thus to obtain a comprehensive picture of a single-cell molecular phenotype. Very sophisticated and sensitive methods for the detection of RNA combined with RNA amplification allow the detection of even low-abundance RNA species [92]. Profiling of single CTCs is promising in shedding new light in the identification and therapeutic targeting of the subpopulations of cells in the primary tumor tissues which are responsible for metastases. Phenotyping the primary tumor alone is not enough as it clearly appears, e.g., considering the discordances of *HER2* expression between tumor tissues and corresponding CTCs which could lead to inefficient treatments [93, 94]. Moreover, the heterogeneity of CTCs is not only evident between different patients but in the blood sample of a single patient as well [61].

A variety of workflows are used for single-cell analysis, but most studies so far are based on the combination of the CellSearch® and DEPArray™ systems followed by WGA and NGS. Using this workflow, a remarkable inter- and intra-patient heterogeneity in the mutational status of CTCs was presented [95] especially in *PIK3CA* mutations [96]. Moreover, in single cells from metastatic triple-negative BrCa patients the presence of different CTC subclones was shown through *TP53* analysis [97]. Polzer et al. using in addition qPCR and aCGH highlighted the correlation of heterogeneity between primary tumors and CTCs, and therapy resistance [98].

The MagSweeper has also been used as the initial step for CTC isolation intended for single-cell analysis. Powell et al. have shown a great heterogeneity in individual CTCs from BrCa patients through gene expression analysis [99]. A mutational heterogeneity between CTCs and tissue tumor cells, and in isolated CTCs of the same patient at different time points, was observed when sequencing exons 9 and 20 of *PIK3CA* [100].

A summary of studies on single-cell analysis in CTCs is presented in Table 3.3.

Table 3.3 Molecular characterization of CTCs based on single-cell analysis in metastatic BrCa patients

Author	Methods			Results
	CTC isolation	Single cell isolation/detection	Molecular characterization	
Polzer et al. [98]	CellSearch®	DEPArray™	WGA, NGS, qPCR, aCGH	Correlation of heterogeneity between primary tumors and CTCs, and therapy resistance
De Luca et al. [95]	CellSearch®	DEPArray™	WGA, NGS	Heterogeneity in the mutational status of CTCs
Pestrin et al. [96]	CellSearch®	DEPArray™	WGA, NGS	Heterogeneity in the *PIK3CA* mutational status of CTCs
Fernandez et al. [97]	CellSearch®	DEPArray™	WGA, NGS	CTC subclones through *TP53* analysis
Shaw et al. [134]	CellSearch®	DEPArray™	WGA, NGS, ddPCR	Mutational intra-heterogeneity in *PIK3CA, TP53, ESR1*, and *KRAS*, more mutations are detected in cfDNA than in CTCs, and primary tumors
Gasch et al. [135]	CellSearch®	Micromanipulation	FISH, WGA, NGS	Great intra-heterogeneity in *HER2* expression and *PIK3CA* mutational status
Powell et al. [99]	MagSweeper	Micromanipulation	Pre-amplification, BioMark™ qPCR system	Great heterogeneity in individual CTCs
Deng et al. [100]	MagSweeper	Immunostaining	NGS	Mutational intra-heterogeneity in exons 9 and 20 of *PIK3CA* in isolated CTCs at different time points
Eirew et al. [136]	Xenografts	FACS	WGS, qPCR	Clonal tumor expansion through dominant mutation clusters
Yu et al. [137]	HB-chip	Immunofluorescence	RNA-ISH	CTCs and CTM exhibit mesenchymal properties associated with the disease progression
Kanwar et al. [138]	MACS	Laser microdissection	WGA, CNVs	Identification of genomic signatures correlated with dormancy and resistance to chemotherapy
Neves et al. [139]	CellSearch®	Flow cytometry	WGA, qPCR, aCGH	Chromosomal aberrations and *PIK3CA* mutations
Papadaki et al. [140]	Density gradient centrifugation	Ariol®		Correlation of stemness and EMT in CTCs through ALDH1 and Twist detection
Babayan et al. [141]	Density gradient centrifugation	Micromanipulation	WGA, NGS	ER heterogeneity between primary tumors and CTCs but not due to *ESR1* mutations

Quality Control (QC) in CTC Analysis

Considerations on the analytical validation of CTC assays include the pre-analytic variables (e.g., materials used, tubes for specimen collection and handling), analytical variables (e.g., type of analysis, sensitivity, specificity, analytical range, reproducibility, clinical applicability, assay-specific controls and calibration), and post-analytic variables (e.g., inter-laboratory performance). Considerations on the clinical validity of CTC assays include the assay and the disease characteristics [101].

Logistical sampling is facilitated only in the course of controlled studies, thereby providing pretreatment and follow-up samples in a statistically powerful sample size. Progress in the clinical implementation can be achieved only if long-term studies with adequate sample sizes are performed and results obtained from such studies are correlated with DFS/OS and other clinical settings. Although most CTC isolation and detection methods are analytically sensitive and specific, the lack of standardization in CTC detection and characterization hampers the implementation of CTC analysis in clinical routine practice. Moreover, the heterogeneity of CTCs and their low numbers in the bloodstream lead to the collection and accumulation of inconsistent data among independent studies. As the clinical results of CTC analyses largely depend on the detection technology used, there is a need for extensive studies specifically designed to compare the efficacy of different detection methods when used to analyze the same clinical samples [67, 102]. A small number of specific CTC-derived biomarkers could be used to identify the optimal assay technologies. Gold standard technologies are needed for comparisons, based on whether the evaluation is quantitative (enumeration of CTCs) or qualitative (molecular characterization of CTCs). CellSearch® could serve as an anchor in the short term for assessments of newer enumeration assay technologies, building on prior clinical evidence for its predictive and prognostic capability [101] (Fig. 3.1. and Fig. 3.2.).

There is a number of studies comparing CTC detection between the CellSearch® system on the one hand and on the other hand CTC-Chips [53], molecular assays [61, 94, 103–106], and other techniques [107, 108]; according to the results presented in these studies there is in most cases a lack of concordance, signaling the urgent need for cross-validation of findings between laboratories and a universal internal and external QC system for both detecting and enumerating CTCs [67, 109]. The newly formed European consortium **CANCER-ID** (*http://www.cancer-id.eu/*), funded by the Innovative Medicines Initiative (IMI), is currently working on cross-comparison of CTC isolation and detection technologies aiming at the establishment of standard protocols for clinical validation of blood-based biomarkers.

Conclusions

Molecular characterization of CTCs holds considerable promise for the identification of therapeutic targets and resistance mechanisms and for real-time monitoring of the efficacy of systemic therapies in patients with metastatic breast cancer. A variety of state-of-the-art systems are available for CTC isolation, detection, and molecular characterization. Analysis of CTCs at the gene expression, DNA methylation, and DNA mutation level holds considerable promise for an individualized treatment approach for patients with metastatic breast cancer.

References

1. Torre LA, Bray F, Siegel RL et al (2015) Global cancer statistics, 2012. CA Cancer J Clin 65:87–108. doi:10.3322/caac.21262
2. DeSantis CE, Fedewa SA, Goding Sauer A et al (2016) Breast cancer statistics, 2015: convergence of incidence rates between black and white women. CA Cancer J Clin 66:31–42. doi:10.3322/caac.21320
3. Siegel RL, Miller KD, Jemal A (2016) Cancer statistics, 2016. CA Cancer J Clin 66:7–30. doi:10.3322/caac.21332
4. Ashworth TR (1869) A case of cancer in which cells similar to those in the tumours were seen in the blood after death. Aust Med J 14:146–147
5. Allard WJ (2004) Tumor cells circulate in the peripheral blood of all major carcinomas but not in healthy subjects or patients with nonmalignant diseases. Clin Cancer Res 10:6897–6904. doi:10.1158/1078-0432.CCR-04-0378
6. Pantel K, Alix-Panabières C (2010) Circulating tumour cells in cancer patients: challenges and perspectives. Trends Mol Med 16:398–406. doi:10.1016/j.molmed.2010.07.001
7. Lianidou ES, Strati A, Markou A (2014) Circulating tumor cells as promising novel biomarkers in solid cancers. Crit Rev Clin Lab Sci 51:160–171. doi:10.3109/10408363.2014.896316
8. Chang YS, di Tomaso E, McDonald DM et al (2000) Mosaic blood vessels in tumors: frequency of cancer cells in contact with flowing blood. Proc Natl Acad Sci 97:14608–14613. doi:10.1073/pnas.97.26.14608
9. Cristofanilli M, Budd GT, Ellis MJ et al (2004) Circulating tumor cells, disease progression, and survival in metastatic breast cancer. N Engl J Med 351:781–791. doi:10.1056/NEJMoa040766
10. Danila DC, Heller G, Gignac GA et al (2007) Circulating tumor cell number and prognosis in progressive castration-resistant prostate cancer. Clin Cancer Res 13:7053–7058. doi:10.1158/1078-0432.CCR-07-1506
11. Shaffer DR, Leversha MA, Danila DC et al (2007) Circulating tumor cell analysis in patients with progressive castration-resistant prostate cancer. Clin Cancer Res 13:2023–2029. doi:10.1158/1078-0432.CCR-06-2701
12. Cohen SJ, Punt CJA, Iannotti N et al (2008) Relationship of circulating tumor cells to tumor response, progression-free survival, and overall survival in patients with metastatic colorectal cancer. J Clin Oncol 26:3213–3221. doi:10.1200/JCO.2007.15.8923
13. Mazel M, Jacot W, Pantel K et al (2015) Frequent expression of PD-L1 on circulating breast cancer cells. Mol Oncol 9:1773–1782. doi:10.1016/j.molonc.2015.05.009
14. Ignatiadis M, Riethdorf S, Bidard F-C et al (2014) International study on inter-reader variability for circulating tumor cells in breast cancer. Breast Cancer Res 16:R43. doi:10.1186/bcr3647
15. Todenhofer T, Hennenlotter J, Feyerabend S et al (2012) Preliminary experience on the use of the Adnatest(R) system for detection of circulating tumor cells in prostate cancer patients. Anticancer Res 32:3507–3513
16. Raimondi C, Nicolazzo C, Gradilone A et al (2014) Circulating tumor cells: exploring intratumor heterogeneity of colorectal cancer. Cancer Biol Ther 15:496. doi:10.4161/cbt.28020
17. Aktas B, Tewes M, Fehm T et al (2009) Stem cell and epithelial-mesenchymal transition markers are frequently overexpressed in circulating tumor cells of metastatic breast cancer patients. Breast Cancer Res 11:R46. doi:10.1186/bcr2333

18. Kasimir-Bauer S, Hoffmann O, Wallwiener D et al (2012) Expression of stem cell and epithelial-mesenchymal transition markers in primary breast cancer patients with circulating tumor cells. Breast Cancer Res 14:R15. doi:10.1186/bcr3099

19. Tewes M, Aktas B, Welt A et al (2009) Molecular profiling and predictive value of circulating tumor cells in patients with metastatic breast cancer: an option for monitoring response to breast cancer related therapies. Breast Cancer Res Treat 115:581–590. doi:10.1007/s10549-008-0143-x

20. Talasaz AH, Powell AA, Huber DE et al (2009) Isolating highly enriched populations of circulating epithelial cells and other rare cells from blood using a magnetic sweeper device. Proc Natl Acad Sci 106:3970–3975. doi:10.1073/pnas.0813188106

21. Nagrath S, Sequist LV, Maheswaran S et al (2007) Isolation of rare circulating tumour cells in cancer patients by microchip technology. Nature 450:1235–1239. doi:10.1038/nature06385

22. Stott SL, Hsu C-H, Tsukrov DI et al (2010) Isolation of circulating tumor cells using a microvortex-generating herringbone-chip. Proc Natl Acad Sci U S A 107:18392–18397. doi:10.1073/pnas.1012539107

23. Ozkumur E, Shah AM, Ciciliano JC et al (2013) Inertial focusing for tumor antigen-dependent and -independent sorting of rare circulating tumor cells. Sci Transl Med 5:179ra47. doi:10.1126/scitranslmed.3005616

24. Kirby BJ, Jodari M, Loftus MS et al (2012) Functional characterization of circulating tumor cells with a prostate-cancer-specific microfluidic device. PLoS One 7:e35976. doi:10.1371/journal.pone.0035976

25. Saucedo-Zeni N, Mewes S, Niestroj R et al (2012) A novel method for the in vivo isolation of circulating tumor cells from peripheral blood of cancer patients using a functionalized and structured medical wire. Int J Oncol 41:1241–1250. doi:10.3892/ijo.2012.1557

26. Ferreira MM, Ramani VC, Jeffrey SS (2016) Circulating tumor cell technologies. Mol Oncol 10:374–394. doi:10.1016/j.molonc.2016.01.007

27. Harouaka RA, Nisic M, Zheng S-Y (2013) Circulating tumor cell enrichment based on physical properties. J Lab Autom 18:455–468. doi:10.1177/2211068213494391

28. Wang L, Asghar W, Demirci U, Wan Y (2013) Nanostructured substrates for isolation of circulating tumor cells. Nano Today 8:347–387

29. Vona G, Sabile A, Louha M et al (2000) Isolation by size of epithelial tumor cells: a new method for the immunomorphological and molecular characterization of circulating tumor cells. Am J Pathol 156:57. doi:10.1016/s0002-9440(10)64706-2

30. Desitter I, Guerrouahen BS, Benali-Furet N et al (2011) A new device for rapid isolation by size and characterization of rare circulating tumor cells. Anticancer Res 31:427–441

31. Chudziak J, Burt DJ, Mohan S et al (2016) Clinical evaluation of a novel microfluidic device for epitope-independent enrichment of circulating tumour cells in patients with small cell lung cancer. Analyst 141:669–678. doi:10.1039/C5AN02156A

32. Rosenberg R, Gertler R, Friederichs J et al (2002) Comparison of two density gradient centrifugation systems for the enrichment of disseminated tumor cells in blood. Cytometry 49:150–158. doi:10.1002/cyto.10161

33. Naume B, Borgen E, Tøssvik S et al (1992) Detection of isolated tumor cells in peripheral blood and in BM: evaluation of a new enrichment method. Cytotherapy 6:244–252. doi:10.1080/14653240410006086

34. Fabbri F, Carloni S, Zoli W et al (2013) Detection and recovery of circulating colon cancer cells using a dielectrophoresis-based device: KRAS mutation status in pure CTCs. Cancer Lett 335:225–231. doi:10.1016/j.canlet.2013.02.015

35. Krivacic RT, Ladanyi A, Curry DN et al (2004) A rare-cell detector for cancer. Proc Natl Acad Sci 101:10501–10504. doi:10.1073/pnas.0404036101

36. Hillig T, Horn P, Nygaard A-B et al (2015) In vitro detection of circulating tumor cells compared by the CytoTrack and CellSearch methods. Tumor Biol 36:4597–4601. doi:10.1007/s13277-015-3105-z

37. Galanzha E, Zharov V (2013) Circulating tumor cell detection and capture by photoacoustic flow cytometry in vivo and ex vivo. Cancers (Basel) 5:1691–1738. doi:10.3390/cancers5041691

38. Alix-Panabières C, Brouillet J-P, Fabbro M et al (2005) Characterization and enumeration of cells secreting tumor markers in the peripheral blood of breast cancer patients. J Immunol Methods 299:177–188. doi:10.1016/j.jim.2005.02.007

39. Alix-Panabières C, Vendrell J-P, Slijper M et al (2009) Full-length cytokeratin-19 is released by human tumor cells: a potential role in metastatic progression of breast cancer. Breast Cancer Res 11:R39. doi:10.1186/bcr2326

40. Alix-Panabières C, Rebillard X, Brouillet J-P et al (2005) Detection of circulating prostate-specific antigen-secreting cells in prostate cancer patients. Clin Chem 51:1538–1541. doi:10.1373/clinchem.2005.049445

41. Alix-Panabières C, Vendrell J-P, Pellé O et al (2007) Detection and characterization of putative metastatic precursor cells in cancer patients. Clin Chem 53:537–539. doi:10.1373/clinchem.2006.079509

42. Denève E, Riethdorf S, Ramos J et al (2013) Capture of viable circulating tumor cells in the liver of colorectal cancer patients. Clin Chem 59:1384–1392. doi:10.1373/clinchem.2013.202846

43. Hodgkinson CL, Morrow CJ, Li Y et al (2014) Tumorigenicity and genetic profiling of circulating tumor cells in small-cell lung cancer. Nat Med 20:897–903. doi:10.1038/nm.3600

44. Baccelli I, Schneeweiss A, Riethdorf S et al (2013) Identification of a population of blood circulating tumor cells from breast cancer patients that initiates metastasis in a xenograft assay. Nat Biotechnol 31:539–544. doi:10.1038/nbt.2576

45. Hou J-M, Krebs MG, Lancashire L et al (2012) Clinical significance and molecular characteristics of circulating tumor cells and circulating tumor microemboli in patients with small-cell lung cancer. J Clin Oncol 30:525–532. doi:10.1200/JCO.2010.33.3716

46. Rossi E, Rugge M, Facchinetti A et al (2014) Retaining the long-survive capacity of Circulating Tumor Cells (CTCs) followed by xeno-transplantation: not only from metastatic cancer of the breast but also of prostate cancer patients. Oncoscience 1:49–56. doi:10.18632/oncoscience.8

47. Stoecklein NH, Fischer JC, Niederacher D, Terstappen LWMM (2016) Challenges for CTC-based liquid biopsies: low CTC frequency and diagnostic leukapheresis as a potential solution. Expert Rev Mol Diagn 16:147–164. doi:10.1586/14737159.2016.1123095

48. Ignatiadis M, Lee M, Jeffrey SS (2015) Circulating tumor cells and circulating tumor DNA: challenges and opportunities on the path to clinical utility. Clin Cancer Res 21:4786–4800. doi:10.1158/1078-0432.CCR-14-1190

49. Hayes DF, Cristofanilli M, Budd GT et al (2006) Circulating tumor cells at each follow-up time point during therapy of metastatic breast cancer patients predict progression-free and overall survival. Clin Cancer Res 12:4218–4224. doi:10.1158/1078-0432.CCR-05-2821

50. Bidard F-C, Peeters DJ, Fehm T et al (2014) Clinical validity of circulating tumour cells in patients with metastatic breast cancer: a pooled analysis of individual patient data. Lancet Oncol 15:406–414. doi:10.1016/S1470-2045(14)70069-5

51. Smerage JB, Barlow WE, Hortobagyi GN et al (2014) Circulating tumor cells and response to chemotherapy in metastatic breast cancer: SWOG S0500. J Clin Oncol 32:3483–3489. doi:10.1200/JCO.2014.56.2561

52. Pestrin M, Bessi S, Galardi F et al (2009) Correlation of HER2 status between primary tumors and corresponding circulating tumor cells in advanced breast cancer patients. Breast Cancer Res Treat 118:523–530. doi:10.1007/s10549-009-0461-7

53. Punnoose EA, Atwal SK, Spoerke JM et al (2010) Molecular biomarker analyses using circulating tumor cells. PLoS One 5:e12517. doi:10.1371/journal.pone.0012517

54. Pestrin M, Bessi S, Puglisi F et al (2012) Final results of a multicenter phase II clinical trial evaluating the activity of single-agent lapatinib in patients with HER2-negative metastatic breast cancer and HER2-positive circulating tumor cells. A proof-of-concept study. Breast Cancer Res Treat 134:283–289. doi:10.1007/s10549-012-2045-1

55. Agelaki S, Kalykaki A, Markomanolaki H et al (2015) Efficacy of Lapatinib in Therapy-Resistant HER2-Positive Circulating Tumor Cells in Metastatic Breast Cancer. PLoS One 10:e0123683. doi:10.1371/journal.pone.0123683

56. Stebbing J, Payne R, Reise J et al (2013) The efficacy of lapatinib in metastatic breast cancer with HER2 non-amplified primary tumors and EGFR positive circulating tumor cells: a proof-of-concept study. PLoS One 8:e62543. doi:10.1371/journal.pone.0062543

57. Kalykaki A, Agelaki S, Kallergi G et al (2014) Elimination of EGFR-expressing circulating tumor cells in patients with metastatic breast cancer treated with gefitinib. Cancer Chemother Pharmacol 73:685–693. doi:10.1007/s00280-014-2387-y

58. Bidard F-C, Fehm T, Ignatiadis M et al (2013) Clinical application of circulating tumor cells in breast cancer: overview of the current interventional trials. Cancer Metastasis Rev 32:179–188. doi:10.1007/s10555-012-9398-0

59. Bidard F-C, Proudhon C, Pierga J-Y (2016) Circulating tumor cells in breast cancer. Mol Oncol 10:418–430. doi:10.1016/j.molonc.2016.01.001

60. Czyż ZT, Hoffmann M, Schlimok G et al (2014) Reliable single cell array CGH for clinical samples. PLoS One 9:e85907. doi:10.1371/journal.pone.0085907

61. Strati A, Markou A, Parisi C et al (2011) Gene expression profile of circulating tumor cells in breast cancer by RT-qPCR. BMC Cancer 11:422. doi:10.1186/1471-2407-11-422

62. Mego M, Mani S A, Lee B-N, et al. (2012) Expression of epithelial-mesenchymal transition-inducing transcription factors in primary breast cancer: the effect of neoadjuvant therapy. Int J Cancer 130:808–816. doi: 10.1002/ijc.26037

63. Joosse SA, Hannemann J, Spotter J et al (2012) Changes in keratin expression during metastatic progression of breast cancer: impact on the detection of circulating tumor cells. Clin Cancer Res 18:993–1003. doi:10.1158/1078-0432.CCR-11-2100

64. Georgoulias V, Bozionelou V, Agelaki S et al (2012) Trastuzumab decreases the incidence of clinical relapses in patients with early breast cancer presenting chemotherapy-resistant CK-19mRNA-positive circulating tumor cells: results of a randomized phase II study. Ann Oncol 23:1744–1750. doi:10.1093/annonc/mds020

65. Bozionellou V, Mavroudis D, Perraki M et al (2004) Trastuzumab administration can effectively target chemotherapy-resistant cytokeratin-19 messenger RNA-positive tumor cells in the peripheral blood and bone marrow of patients with breast cancer. Clin Cancer Res 10:8185–8194. doi:10.1158/1078-0432.CCR-03-0094

66. Lowes L, Allan A (2014) Recent advances in the molecular characterization of circulating tumor cells. Cancers (Basel) 6:595–624. doi:10.3390/cancers6010595

67. Lianidou ES, Markou A (2011) Circulating tumor cells in breast cancer: detection systems, molecular characterization, and future challenges. Clin Chem 57:1242–1255. doi:10.1373/clinchem.2011.165068

68. Sieuwerts AM, Kraan J, Bolt-de Vries J et al (2009) Molecular characterization of circulating tumor cells in large quantities of contaminating leukocytes by a multiplex real-time PCR. Breast Cancer Res Treat 118:455–468. doi:10.1007/s10549-008-0290-0

69. Aktas B, Kasimir-Bauer S, Heubner M et al (2011) Molecular profiling and prognostic relevance of circulating tumor cells in the blood of ovarian cancer patients at primary diagnosis and after platinum-based chemotherapy. Int J Gynecol Cancer 21:822–830. doi:10.1097/IGC.0b013e318216cb91

70. Rödiger S, Liebsch C, Schmidt C et al (2014) Nucleic acid detection based on the use of microbeads: a review. Microchim Acta 181:1151–1168. doi:10.1007/s00604-014-1243-4

71. Markou A, Strati A, Malamos N et al (2011) Molecular characterization of circulating tumor cells in breast cancer by a liquid bead array hybridization assay. Clin Chem 57:421–430. doi:10.1373/clinchem.2010.154328

72. Parisi C, Markou A, Strati A, Lianidou E (2013) Abstract 1462: development of a multiplexed RT-PCR-coupled liquid bead array assay for the molecular characterization of CTCs. Cancer Res 73:1462–1462. doi:10.1158/1538-7445.AM2013-1462

73. Androulakis N, Agelaki S, Perraki M et al (2012) Clinical relevance of circulating CK-19mRNA-positive tumour cells before front-line treatment in patients with metastatic breast cancer. Br J Cancer 106:1917–1925. doi:10.1038/bjc.2012.202

74. Ramirez J-M, Fehm T, Orsini M et al (2014) Prognostic relevance of viable circulating tumor cells detected by EPISPOT in metastatic breast cancer patients. Clin Chem 60:214–221. doi:10.1373/clinchem.2013.215079

75. Schneck H, Blassl C, Meier-Stiegen F et al (2013) Analysing the mutational status of PIK3CA in circulating tumor cells from metastatic breast cancer patients. Mol Oncol 7:976–986. doi:10.1016/j.molonc.2013.07.007

76. Markou A, Farkona S, Schiza C et al (2014) PIK3CA mutational status in circulating tumor cells can change during disease recurrence or progression in patients with breast cancer. Clin Cancer Res 20:5823–5834. doi:10.1158/1078-0432.CCR-14-0149

77. Pixberg C, Schulz W, Stoecklein N, Neves R (2015) Characterization of DNA methylation in circulating tumor cells. Genes (Basel) 6:1053–1075. doi:10.3390/genes6041053

78. Abrahamson M, Alvarez-Fernandez M, Nathanson C-M (2003) Cystatins. Biochem Soc Symp:179–199

79. Stenman G, Aström AK, Röijer E et al (1997) Assignment of a novel cysteine proteinase inhibitor (CST6) to 11q13 by fluorescence in situ hybridization. Cytogenet Cell Genet 76:45–46

80. Ai L, Kim W-J, Kim T-Y et al (2006) Epigenetic silencing of the tumor suppressor cystatin M occurs during breast cancer progression. Cancer Res 66:7899–7909. doi:10.1158/0008-5472.CAN-06-0576

81. Chimonidou M, Strati A, Tzitzira A et al (2011) DNA methylation of tumor suppressor and metastasis suppressor genes in circulating tumor cells. Clin Chem 57:1169–1177. doi:10.1373/clinchem.2011.165902

82. Hurst DR (2012) Metastasis suppression by BRMS1 associated with SIN3 chromatin remodeling complexes. Cancer Metastasis Rev 31:641–651. doi:10.1007/s10555-012-9363-y

83. Hurst DR, Edmonds MD, Scott GK et al (2009) Breast cancer metastasis suppressor 1 upregulates miR-146, which suppresses breast cancer metastasis. Cancer Res 69:1279–1283. doi:10.1158/0008-5472.CAN-08-3559

84. Cicek M (2005) Breast cancer metastasis suppressor 1 inhibits gene expression by targeting nuclear factor- B activity. Cancer Res 65:3586–3595. doi:10.1158/0008-5472.CAN-04-3139

85. Vaidya KS, Harihar S, Phadke PA et al (2008) Breast cancer metastasis suppressor-1 differentially modulates growth factor signaling. J Biol Chem 283:28354–28360. doi:10.1074/jbc.M710068200

86. Balgkouranidou I, Chimonidou M, Milaki G et al (2014) Breast cancer metastasis suppressor-1 promoter methylation in cell-free DNA provides prognostic information in non-small cell lung cancer. Br J Cancer 110:2054–2062. doi:10.1038/bjc.2014.104

87. Lefebvre V, Dumitriu B, Penzo-Méndez A et al (2007) Control of cell fate and differentiation by Sry-related high-mobility-group box (Sox) transcription factors. Int J Biochem Cell Biol 39:2195–2214. doi:10.1016/j.biocel.2007.05.019

88. Zhang W, Glöckner SC, Guo M et al (2008) Epigenetic inactivation of the canonical Wnt antagonist SRY-box containing gene 17 in colorectal cancer. Cancer Res 68:2764–2772. doi:10.1158/0008-5472.CAN-07-6349

89. Fu D-Y, Wang Z-M, Li-Chen, et al. (2010) Sox17, the canonical Wnt antagonist, is epigenetically inactivated by promoter methylation in human breast cancer. Breast Cancer Res Treat 119:601–612. doi: 10.1007/s10549-009-0339-8

90. Chimonidou M, Strati A, Malamos N et al (2013) SOX17 promoter methylation in circulating tumor cells and matched cell-free DNA isolated from plasma of patients with breast cancer. Clin Chem 59:270–279. doi:10.1373/clinchem.2012.191551

91. Parisi C, Mastoraki S, Markou A et al (2016) Development and validation of a multiplex methylation specific PCR-coupled liquid bead array for liquid biopsy analysis. Clin Chim Acta 461:156–164. doi:10.1016/j.cca.2016.08.003

92. Galler K, Bräutigam K, Große C et al (2014) Making a big thing of a small cell—recent advances in single cell analysis. Analyst 139:1237. doi:10.1039/c3an01939j

93. Ignatiadis M, Rothé F, Chaboteaux C et al (2011) HER2-positive circulating tumor cells in breast cancer. PLoS One 6:e15624. doi:10.1371/journal.pone.0015624

94. Fehm T, Müller V, Aktas B et al (2010) HER2 status of circulating tumor cells in patients with metastatic breast cancer: a prospective, multicenter trial. Breast Cancer Res Treat 124:403–412. doi:10.1007/s10549-010-1163-x

95. De Luca F, Rotunno G, Salvianti F et al (2016) Mutational analysis of single circulating tumor cells by next generation sequencing in metastatic breast cancer. Oncotarget 7(18):26107–26119. doi:10.18632/oncotarget.8431

96. Pestrin M, Salvianti F, Galardi F et al (2015) Heterogeneity of PIK3CA mutational status at the single cell level in circulating tumor cells from metastatic breast cancer patients. Mol Oncol 9:749–757. doi:10.1016/j.molonc.2014.12.001

97. Fernandez SV, Bingham C, Fittipaldi P et al (2014) TP53 mutations detected in circulating tumor cells present in the blood of metastatic triple negative breast cancer patients. Breast Cancer Res 16:445. doi:10.1186/s13058-014-0445-3

98. Polzer B, Medoro G, Pasch S et al (2014) Molecular profiling of single circulating tumor cells with diagnostic intention. EMBO Mol Med 6:1371–1386. doi:10.15252/emmm. 201404033

99. Powell AA, Talasaz AH, Zhang H et al (2012) Single cell profiling of circulating tumor cells: transcriptional heterogeneity and diversity from breast cancer cell lines. PLoS One 7:e33788. doi:10.1371/journal.pone.0033788

100. Deng G, Krishnakumar S, Powell AA et al (2014) Single cell mutational analysis of PIK3CA in circulating tumor cells and metastases in breast cancer reveals heterogeneity, discordance, and mutation persistence in cultured disseminated tumor cells from bone marrow. BMC Cancer 14:456. doi:10.1186/1471-2407-14-456

101. Parkinson DR, Dracopoli N, Gumbs Petty B et al (2012) Considerations in the development of circulating tumor cell technology for clinical use. J Transl Med 10:138. doi:10.1186/1479-5876-10-138

102. Lianidou ES, Markou A, Strati A (2015) The role of CTCs as tumor biomarkers. Adv Exp Med Biol 867:341–367. doi:10.1007/978-94-017-7215-0_21

103. Andreopoulou E, Yang L-Y, Rangel KM et al (2012) Comparison of assay methods for detection of circulating tumor cells in metastatic breast cancer: adnagen AdnaTest BreastCancer Select/Detect™ versus Veridex CellSearch™ system. Int J Cancer 130:1590–1597. doi:10.1002/ijc.26111

104. Van der Auwera I, Peeters D, Benoy IH et al (2010) Circulating tumour cell detection: a direct comparison between the CellSearch System, the AdnaTest and CK-19/mammaglobin RT-PCR in patients with metastatic breast cancer. Br J Cancer 102:276–284. doi:10.1038/sj.bjc.6605472

105. Müller V, Riethdorf S, Rack B et al (2012) Prognostic impact of circulating tumor cells assessed with the CellSearch System™ and AdnaTest Breast™ in metastatic breast cancer patients: the DETECT study. Breast Cancer Res 14:R118. doi:10.1186/bcr3243

106. Guo W, Yang X-R, Sun Y-F et al (2014) Clinical significance of EpCAM mRNA-positive circulating tumor cells in hepatocellular carcinoma by an optimized negative enrichment and qRT-PCR-based platform. Clin Cancer Res 20:4794–4805. doi:10.1158/1078-0432. CCR-14-0251

107. Massard C, Oulhen M, Le Moulec S et al (2016) Phenotypic and genetic heterogeneity of tumor tissue and circulating tumor cells in patients with metastatic castrationresistant prostate cancer: a report from the PETRUS prospective study. Oncotarget. doi:10.18632/oncotarget.10396

108. Pantel K, Denève E, Nocca D et al (2012) Circulating epithelial cells in patients with benign colon diseases. Clin Chem 58:936–940. doi:10.1373/clinchem.2011.175570

109. Lianidou ES (2012) Circulating tumor cells—New challenges ahead. Clin Chem 58:805–807. doi:10.1373/clinchem.2011.180646

110. Lianidou ES, Markou A (2011) Circulating tumor cells as emerging tumor biomarkers in breast cancer. Clin Chem Lab Med 49:1579–1590. doi:10.1515/CCLM.2011.628

111. Banys M, Müller V, Melcher C et al (2013) Circulating tumor cells in breast cancer. Clin Chim Acta 423:39–45. doi:10.1016/j.cca.2013.03.029

112. Cristofanilli M (2005) Circulating tumor cells: a novel prognostic factor for newly diagnosed metastatic breast cancer. J Clin Oncol 23:1420–1430. doi:10.1200/JCO.2005.08.140

113. De Giorgi U, Valero V, Rohren E et al (2010) Circulating tumor cells and bone metastases as detected by FDG-PET/CT in patients with metastatic breast cancer. Ann Oncol 21:33–39. doi:10.1093/annonc/mdp262

114. Budd GT, Cristofanilli M, Ellis MJ et al (2006) Circulating tumor cells versus imaging—Predicting overall survival in metastatic breast cancer. Clin Cancer Res 12:6403–6409. doi:10.1158/1078-0432.CCR-05-1769

115. Giordano A, Giuliano M, De Laurentiis M et al (2012) Circulating tumor cells in immunohistochemical subtypes of metastatic breast cancer: lack of prediction in HER2-positive disease treated with targeted therapy. Ann Oncol 23:1144–1150. doi:10.1093/annonc/mdr434

116. Wallwiener M, Hartkopf AD, Baccelli I et al (2013) The prognostic impact of circulating tumor cells in subtypes of metastatic breast cancer. Breast Cancer Res Treat 137:503–510. doi:10.1007/s10549-012-2382-0

117. Pierga JY, Hajage D, Bachelot T et al (2012) High independent prognostic and predictive value of circulating tumor cells compared with serum tumor markers in a large prospective trial in first-line chemotherapy for metastatic breast cancer patients. Ann Oncol 23:618–624. doi:10.1093/annonc/mdr263

118. Giuliano M, Giordano A, Jackson S et al (2011) Circulating tumor cells as prognostic and predictive markers in metastatic breast cancer patients receiving first-line systemic treatment. Breast Cancer Res 13:R67. doi:10.1186/bcr2907

119. Nakamura S, Yagata H, Ohno S et al (2010) Multi-center study evaluating circulating tumor cells as a surrogate for response to treatment and overall survival in metastatic breast cancer. Breast Cancer 17:199–204. doi:10.1007/s12282-009-0139-3

120. Nole F, Munzone E, Zorzino L et al (2008) Variation of circulating tumor cell levels during treatment of metastatic breast cancer: prognostic and therapeutic implications. Ann Oncol 19:891–897. doi:10.1093/annonc/mdm558

121. Liu JF, Kindelberger D, Doyle C et al (2013) Predictive value of circulating tumor cells (CTCs) in newly-diagnosed and recurrent ovarian cancer patients. Gynecol Oncol 131:352–356. doi:10.1016/j.ygyno.2013.08.006

122. Munzone E, Nolé F, Goldhirsch A et al (2010) Changes of HER2 Status in Circulating Tumor Cells Compared With the Primary Tumor During Treatment for Advanced Breast Cancer. Clinical Breast Cancer 10:392–397. doi:10.3816/CBC.2010.n.052

123. Sieuwerts AM, Jeffrey SS (2012) Multiplex molecular analysis of CTCs. Recent Results Cancer Res 195:125–140. doi:10.1007/978-3-642-28160-0_11

124. Reinholz MM, Kitzmann KA, Tenner K et al (2011) Cytokeratin-19 and Mammaglobin Gene Expression in Circulating Tumor Cells from Metastatic Breast Cancer Patients Enrolled in North Central Cancer Treatment Group Trials, N0234/336/436/437. Clin Cancer Res 17:7183–7193. doi:10.1158/1078-0432.CCR-11-0981

125. Benoy IH, Elst H, Philips M et al (2006) Real-time RT–PCR detection of disseminated tumour cells in bone marrow has superior prognostic significance in comparison with circulating tumour cells in patients with breast cancer. Br J Cancer 94:672–680. doi:10.1038/sj.bjc.6602985

126. Pierga J-Y, Bidard F-C, Denis MG, de Cremoux P (2007) Prognostic value of peripheral blood double detection of CK19 and MUC1 mRNA positive cells detected by RT-quantitative PCR in 94 breast cancer patients with a follow up of 9 years. Mol Oncol 1:267–268. doi:10.1016/j.molonc.2007.09.005

127. Bidard F-C, Vincent-Salomon A, Sigal-Zafrani B et al (2008) Prognosis of women with stage IV breast cancer depends on detection of circulating tumor cells rather than disseminated tumor cells. Ann Oncol 19:496–500. doi:10.1093/annonc/mdm507

128. Li W, O'Shaughnessy JA, Hayes DF et al (2016) Biomarker associations with efficacy of abiraterone acetate and exemestane in postmenopausal patients with estrogen receptor-positive metastatic breast cancer. Clin Cancer Res 22(24):6002–6009. doi:10.1158/1078-0432.CCR-15-2452

129. Sieuwerts AM, Mostert B, Bolt-de Vries J et al (2011) mRNA and microRNA expression profiles in circulating tumor cells and primary tumors of metastatic breast cancer patients. Clin Cancer Res 17:3600–3618. doi:10.1158/1078-0432.CCR-11-0255

130. Meng S, Tripathy D, Shete S et al (2006) uPAR and HER-2 gene status in individual breast cancer cells from blood and tissues. Proc Natl Acad Sci U S A 103:17361–17365. doi:10.1073/pnas.0608113103
131. Kallergi G, Papadaki M a, Politaki E, et al. (2011) Epithelial to mesenchymal transition markers expressed in circulating tumour cells of early and metastatic breast cancer patients. Breast Cancer Res 13:R59. doi: 10.1186/bcr2896
132. Theodoropoulos PA, Polioudaki H, Agelaki S et al (2010) Circulating tumor cells with a putative stem cell phenotype in peripheral blood of patients with breast cancer. Cancer Lett 288:99–106. doi:10.1016/j.canlet.2009.06.027
133. Kallergi G, Markomanolaki H, Giannoukaraki V et al (2009) Hypoxia-inducible factor-1alpha and vascular endothelial growth factor expression in circulating tumor cells of breast cancer patients. Breast Cancer Res 11:R84. doi:10.1186/bcr2452
134. Shaw JA, Guttery DS, Hills A et al (2016) Mutation analysis of cell-free DNA and single circulating tumor cells in metastatic breast cancer patients with high CTC counts. Clin Cancer Res. doi:10.1158/1078-0432.CCR-16-0825
135. Gasch C, Oldopp T, Mauermann O et al (2016) Frequent detection of PIK3CA mutations in single circulating tumor cells of patients suffering from HER2-negative metastatic breast cancer. Mol Oncol 10:1330–1343. doi:10.1016/j.molonc.2016.07.005
136. Eirew P, Steif A, Khattra J et al (2015) Dynamics of genomic clones in breast cancer patient xenografts at single-cell resolution. Nature 518:422–426. doi:10.1038/nature13952
137. Yu M, Bardia A, Wittner BS et al (2013) Circulating breast tumor cells exhibit dynamic changes in epithelial and mesenchymal composition. Science 339:580–584. doi:10.1126/science.1228522
138. Kanwar N, Hu P, Bedard P et al (2015) Identification of genomic signatures in circulating tumor cells from breast cancer. Int J Cancer 137:332–344. doi:10.1002/ijc.29399
139. Neves RPL, Raba K, Schmidt O et al (2014) Genomic high-resolution profiling of single CKpos/CD45neg flow-sorting purified circulating tumor cells from patients with metastatic breast cancer. Clin Chem 60:1290–1297. doi:10.1373/clinchem.2014.222331
140. Papadaki MA, Kallergi G, Zafeiriou Z et al (2014) Co-expression of putative stemness and epithelial-to-mesenchymal transition markers on single circulating tumour cells from patients with early and metastatic breast cancer. BMC Cancer 14:651. doi:10.1186/1471-2407-14-651
141. Babayan A, Hannemann J, Spötter J et al (2013) Heterogeneity of estrogen receptor expression in circulating tumor cells from metastatic breast cancer patients. PLoS One 8:e75038. doi:10.1371/journal.pone.0075038

Chapter 4
Epithelial-Mesenchymal Transition (EMT) and Cancer Stem Cells (CSCs): The Traveling Metastasis

Michal Mego, James Reuben, and Sendurai A. Mani

Abstract The metastatic cascade is a series of biological steps that tumor cells must complete to exit the primary tumor and develop a new tumor at a distant site. Cancer dissemination, which involves circulating tumor cells (CTCs), is a crucial step for metastasis. Recent progress in solid tumor stem cell biology suggests that cells that mediate metastasis are cancer stem cells. Invasive potential of cancer cells is induced by a process known as epithelial to mesenchymal transition (EMT). This biological program is accompanied by loss of cell polarity, cell-cell contacts, and downregulation of epithelial genes accompanied by upregulation of mesenchymal genes. Moreover, EMT is associated with increased cell motility, resistance to chemotherapy, and cancer stem cell phenotype. CTCs are a unique and heterogeneous cell population with established prognostic and predictive value in certain clinical situations. The possibility of collecting sequential blood samples for real-time monitoring of systemic therapy efficacy constitutes new possibilities to evaluate therapies based on the genomic profiling of CTCs and to improve the clinical management of patients by personalized therapy.

Keywords Circulating tumor cells • Epithelial-mesenchymal transition • Cancer stem cells

---

M. Mego (✉)
National Cancer Institute, Klenova 1, Bratislava 833 10, Slovak Republic

Department of Oncology, Faculty of Medicine, Comenius University and National Cancer Institute, Klenova 1, Bratislava 833 10, Slovakia
e-mail: misomego@gmail.com

J. Reuben
Department of Hematopathology, Division of Pathology/Lab Medicine, The University of Texas MD Anderson Cancer Center, Houston, TX, USA

S.A. Mani
Department of Translational Molecular Pathology, Division of Pathology/Lab Medicine, The University of Texas MD Anderson Cancer Center, Houston, TX, USA

© Springer International Publishing AG 2017
M. Cristofanilli (ed.), *Liquid Biopsies in Solid Tumors*, Cancer Drug Discovery and Development, DOI 10.1007/978-3-319-50956-3_4

67

Introduction

Breast cancer is one of the most common cancers in women, with an estimated 231,840 new cases diagnosed and 40,290 deaths in the USA since the beginning of 2015 [1]. Despite advances in the diagnostics and adjuvant therapy, a substantial proportion of women are still diagnosed with metastatic disease either at initial presentation (5–10%) or during the course of treatment (30%) [1]. Metastatic disease is usually an incurable condition; systemic chemotherapies have only palliative effects in vast majority of patients [2]. This failure has been associated with multiple biological mechanisms related to factors including the intrinsic heterogeneity of breast cancer, which enables the classification of breast cancer into molecular subtypes [3–5]. Recent advances in solid tumor stem cell biology suggest that cancer stem cells mediate metastases [6]. Moreover, cancer stem cells isolated from human cancers, including solid tumors as well as hematopoietic malignancies, have been shown to intrinsically possess high resistance to chemotherapy or radiotherapy [7–9].

Metastasis

The metastatic cascade is a series of biological steps that tumor cells must complete to exit the primary tumor and develop a new tumor at a distant site. Tumor cells must invade the basement membrane and surrounding tissue and enter the bloodstream or lymphatics. Tumor cells capable of surviving in the peripheral blood may eventually extravasate the bloodstream, where some of them are capable of establishing a macroscopic tumor. Invasion, the first critical step in the metastatic process, requires changes in cell-cell adhesion as well as cell-matrix interaction. Invasion is further enabled by proteolytic degradation of the extracellular matrix (ECM), which allows cancer cells to penetrate tissue boundaries. Degradation of the ECM is mediated predominately by matrix metalloproteinases (MMPs) and the urokinase plasminogen activator (uPA) system [10]. In fact, a significant proportion of circulating tumor cells (CTCs), detected in patients with advanced stage disease, exhibit amplification of uPA receptor [10]. Invasive potential of cancer cells is induced by a process known as epithelial to mesenchymal transition (EMT). This biological program is accompanied by loss of cell polarity, cell-cell contacts, and downregulation of epithelial genes accompanied by upregulation of mesenchymal genes [11]. Moreover, EMT is associated with increased cell motility, resistance to chemotherapy, and cancer stem cell phenotype [12].

Cancer cells migrate via blood either as a single cell or as a cluster, which is referred to as single-cell migration and collective-cell migration, respectively [13, 14]. Activation of EMT seems to be crucial in mesenchymal-cell migration while activation of Rho GTPases has an important role in amoeboid single-cell migration [14, 15]. Amoeboid-cell migration is characterized by loss of attachment to the

ECM and loss of cell polarity, which results in rapid movement following the path of least resistance. Both induction of EMT and activation of rhoGTPases led to activation of MMPs with further degradation of ECM and increased cancer cell invasion [16, 17]. Collective-cell migration requires continued presentation of intercellular junctions; therefore, in this case, cancer cells invade, intravasate, and disseminate as clusters that are highly efficient at embolizing in lymphatic or blood vessels and surviving in the peripheral circulation [18].

The bloodstream is highly unfavorable to the survival of tumor cells owing to physical shear forces, immune surveillance due to the presence of immune cells, and anoikis, which all contribute to metastatic insufficiency [19–21]. Furthermore, minor perturbations of immune surveillance could purportedly be responsible for controlling tumor dissemination, and favor conducive environment for the survival and dissemination of CTCs, leading to progression of cancer [22]. Upon intravasation, CTCs interact with circulating coagulation factors and platelets via tissue factors (TF), fibrin, and selections to form microemboli. In order to extravasate, CTCs secrete factors that disrupt endothelial cell junctions and increase vascular permeability, thus facilitating transendothelial passage of tumor cells [23].

It is supposed that EMT has a major role in the initial step of the metastatic cascade, where, through EMT, some tumor cells acquire the ability to invade the basement membrane and surrounding stroma and then intravasate. Following extravasation, a process termed mesenchymal to epithelial transition (MET) has been proposed to help tumor cells in the secondary organ to undergo "redifferentiation" to an epithelial phenotype and form metastases with similar histological characteristics as the primary tumor. It is unclear if all disseminated cancer cells undergo MET and lose their mesenchymal and/or cancer stem cell phenotype or if the fraction of mesenchymal and/or cancer stem cells give rise to numerous differentiated progeny during colonization [24]. However, both processes would result in a differentiated, epithelial tumor phenotype.

Moreover, tumor dissemination is also affected by stromal cells, which modulate tumor cell invasion and migration and could serve as pathfinders through the ECM [25]. Fibroblasts and myofibroblasts represent the majority of stromal cells within breast cancer. Carcinoma-associated fibroblasts (CAFs), isolated from invasive human breast tumors, are more competent at promoting the progression of breast cancer cells than comparable cells from outside of the tumor masses [26, 27].

An increasing body of literature suggests that chemokines and their receptors play an important role in cancer progression, migration of cancer cells, and metastasis formation [28–31]. Moreover, chemokines produced at the site of dissemination can dictate whether the disseminated cells will thrive and colonize those organs. Data suggest that along with chemokine gradients in the blood or tumor microenvironment, the "premetastatic niche" that could be formed by bone marrow-derived hematopoietic cells facilitates targeted colonization. These bone marrow-derived cells attract tumor cells as well as propose to support the developing metastases [32, 33].

Role of CSCs in Metastasis

Recent progress in solid tumor stem cell biology suggests that cells that mediate metastasis are cancer stem cells [6]. In breast cancer, markers to identify putative cancer stem cells have been described based on their ability to initiate xenograft tumors in immunocompromised mice. Al-Hajj et al. observed that CD44+/CD24−/lo tumor cells isolated from human breast tumors displayed increased ability to form tumors in the mammary fat pad of NOD/SCID mice. Their study showed that as few as 100 CD44+/CD24−/lo human breast tumor cells are capable of recapitulating the tumors from which they were originally isolated, compared to 10,000 cells of CD44−/low and CD24+ phenotypes failed to form tumors [34]. The tumor-initiating capacity of this population has been further refined in transplant studies reported by Ginestier et al. Their studies examined aldehyde dehydrogenase 1 (ALDH1) activity that is characteristic of hematopoietic stem cells. Using a flow cytometry assay to sort positive ALDH1 activity in human breast tumor cells, they demonstrated that CD44+/CD24− residing in the sub-population of cells within the ALDH1-positive pool possess the tumor outgrowth potential [35].

Role of Complete and Partial EMT in Promoting CSC Properties

A number of studies have shown that carcinoma cells often activate an EMT program to gain the ability and to execute the multiple steps of the invasion–metastasis cascade [36]. During an EMT, epithelial cells lose cell–cell contacts and cell polarity, acquire mesenchymal gene expression, and acquire a mesenchymal appearance due to major changes in their cytoskeleton, which enables the cancer cells to increase motility and invasiveness [37, 38].

There is also a link established between the induction of an EMT in and the acquisition of stem cell markers, which illustrate a direct link between the EMT program and the gain of stem cell properties [12]. Epithelial cells undergoing a complete EMT to become mesenchymal have been shown to possess stem cell properties. Similarly, even cells undergoing partial EMT (hybrid E/M phenotype) also proposed to gain stem cell properties [39]. Mesenchymal cells migrate individually, while hybrid E/M cells move collectively as observed during gastrulation, wound healing, and/or the formation of tumor clusters detected as CTCs [40]. Emerging data suggest that partial EMT, (hybrid E/M) phenotype, need not be "metastable," and strengthen the emerging notion that partial EMT, but not necessarily a complete EMT, is associated with aggressive tumor progression [41].

CTCs and Metastasis

Cancer dissemination, which involves CTCs, is a crucial step for metastasis. CTCs are very rare cells surrounded by billions of hematopoietic cells in the bloodstream. CTCs are supposed to represent a heterogeneous population of cells with different phenotypes and biological value [21]. Metastatic disease is usually a late event during disease progression, and the risk of metastases increases with the size of the primary tumor. However, experimental and clinical data indicate that tumor dissemination via CTCs is a relatively early event during the course of the disease [42–45]. In a transgenic mouse model of breast cancer, disseminated tumor cells were found in the bone marrow and lung tissue at the stage of preinvasive atypical hyperplasia, before individual cells started to break through the basement membrane [42].

The flow of cancer cells from the primary site to the metastatic site may not be unidirectional. It now seems plausible that metastatic tumors can release CTCs, which can then rejoin the original primary tumor, a process termed "self-seeding" [46, 47]. Self-seeding likely requires two distinct functions: the ability of a tumor to attract its own circulating progeny and the ability of CTCs to re-infiltrate the primary tumor. More importantly, these "seeder" cells only colonize to preexisting tumors, not to the intact sites, and thus these cells require little adaptation to grow at already established tumor sites. The concept of self-seeding helps explain some of the clinical observations, such as the local relapse of the tumor following apparently complete removal of breast tumors [47]. It appears that self-seeding is one of the major drivers of tumor progression in solid tumors, and CTCs are mediators of tumor self-seeding [46, 47]. The presence of CTCs in peripheral blood, thus, represents a surrogate marker for tumor self-seeding potential.

It seems that not all CTCs are equally capable of forming metastasis [48, 49]. Clinical observation from patients who had ascitic fluid caused by different cancers, and treated with peritoneovenous shunts to alleviate the symptoms associated with ascites, revealed that ascites fluid infused directly into the jugular vein had carried up to a billion viable tumorigenic cells per week into the systemic circulation for many months. However, follow-up autopsies revealed that (a) some of the patients had no metastasis in any organ, (b) some other patients had small multiple tumor deposits in many organs, and (c) some patients had even more metastases in the same organs in which metastases were already present. Interestingly, none of these patients suffered any symptoms from these tumor deposits and all died because of advancing growth of their originally inoperable tumor [50]. These data support the concept of heterogeneity of CTCs with their capabilities of initiating and forming different metastases.

Recently, the existence and phenotype of metastasis-initiating cells (MICs) among CTCs have been experimentally demonstrated in a xenograft assay in breast cancer. It was shown that MIC-containing CTC populations expressed EPCAM, CD44, CD47, and c-MET. In a small cohort of patients with metastases, the number of EPCAM(+)CD44(+)CD47(+)MET(+) CTCs, but not the bulk EPCAM(+) CTCs, correlated with lower overall survival and increased number of metastatic sites [45].

CTC with Complete and Partial EMT in Metastasis

Experimental and clinical data suggest a close relationship between activation of EMT program and generation of CTCs [51–54]. EMT is associated with a set of molecular changes in epithelial cancer cells that results in increased motility and induction of proteases that are involved in degradation of the ECM, facilitating thus invasion and intravasation into the bloodstream [55, 56]. EMT has also been linked to the stem cell phenotype and resistance to apoptotic signals, facilitating EMT-derived CTCs to survive in foreign environments [12]. EMT is closely linked to immunity and activation of EMT program induces T-regulatory cells and impaired dendritic cells, suggesting an immunosuppressive effect of EMT that might support cancer dissemination mediated by CTCs [19, 20, 57]. Moreover, epithelial cells that are undergoing EMT program rarely shed all of their preexisting epithelial features; therefore, EMT usually produces cells with a spectrum of intermediate epithelial and mesenchymal phenotypic states. In fact, a recent paper shows that subpopulations of CTCs have partial or complete EMT phenotype [51–54]. This association suggests that EMT pathways facilitate both the "generation" and "maintenance" of CTCs, as well as the fact that EMT-derived CTCs that are more adept at colonizing distant sites [21]. EMT participates in the induction of the angiogenic switch, favoring the growth of new vessels and thus facilitating survival of CTCs after extravasation and in the colonization of new microenvironments [58, 59]. EMT is associated with upregulation of cell-to-cell adhesion molecules mediating adhesion of cancer cells to the endothelium and enhanced capacity to migrate through an endothelial monolayer in vitro that also contribute to intra- and extravasation [60, 61]. EMT is associated with EGFR-induced tissue factor expression. Increased expression of tissue factor may further facilitate the formation of tumor emboli and arrest in the capillary bed. These data suggest an important role for EMT in different features of CTC biology [62].

Inhibiting the expression of the EMT-inducing transcription factor, TWIST, in a highly metastatic 4T1 murine mammary cell line reduced metastatic burden and the number of CTCs in mice bearing xenograft tumor [63]. In mice, subcutaneous injection of transformed hamster oral keratinocytes expressing either vector or a downstream effector of the TGF-β pathway (p12CKD2–aP1) and exhibiting the EMT phenotype formed tumors similarly, but only EMT-induced cells were detected in the bloodstream. However, neither cell type was able to form lung metastases. By contrast, after intravenous inoculation, only mice injected with non-EMT (control) cells developed lung metastases [49]. In another experiment parenteral bladder cancer cell line with EMT characteristics formed lung metastases after injection into the mouse bladder in contrast to a more epithelial daughter cell line isolated from bone metastasis via in vivo selection. Interestingly, after intracardiac injection, the epithelial cell line developed more overt lung metastasis than the mesenchymal one [48]. Using a spontaneous squamous cell carcinoma mouse model, Tsai et al. showed that activation of Twist1, the EMT-inducing transcription factor, is sufficient to promote carcinoma cells to undergo EMT and disseminate into blood circulation. In distant sites, turning off Twist1 allows reversion of EMT and it is essential for disseminated tumor cells to proliferate and form metastases [64]. It seems that EMT facilitates intravasation and generation of CTCs; however, EMT-derived cells are less competent at forming overt metastasis. By contrast, epithelial cells have probably more limited capacity for active intravasation, but they are more prone to grow in secondary organs [55, 65].

Several translational studies demonstrated activation of EMT in a subpopulation of CTCs including expression of EMT-inducing transcription factors on CTCs [51–54]. However, there was no correlation even between CTCs with EMT phenotype and expression of EMT transcription factors in tumor tissue [66]. Transient, dynamic, and reversible characteristics of EMT process limit detection of EMT within primary tumor tissues [67]. In the study by Aktas et al. several EMT-associated markers (TWIST1, AKT2, and PI3Kα) were detected on CTCs using a reverse transcription (RT-PCR)-based assay and this study demonstrated that at least one of the EMT markers were expressed in 62% of the CTCs [68]. In another study, it was shown that phosphorylated EGFR, HIF1α, HER2, and PI3K/Akt signaling kinases that can regulate EMT are present in CTCs [69–72]. However, these studies used epithelial markers for the detection of CTCs, which suggest that CTCs with partial or complete EMT phenotype might have been missed from this analysis. EMT is associated with the acquisition of cancer-stem cell properties, and several studies showed that CTCs express markers linked to cancer stem cells including NOTCH1 and ALDH1 [68, 73, 74].

Serial monitoring of CTCs in 11 patients over a period of time suggested a strong association of appearance of mesenchymal CTCs with disease progression. In addition, in response to therapy and disease progression, patients displayed reversible shifts between mesenchymal and epithelial CTC state. Moreover, mesenchymal CTCs were observed in as both single cells and multicellular clusters, expressing known EMT regulators [54]. These data reinstate the role for EMT in the blood-borne dissemination of human breast cancer [54]. These data advocate that there is a continuum in the development of CTC phenotypes ranging from epithelial differentiation to mesenchymal phenotype, including those with a partial EMT phenotype. Moreover, these data also postulate the idea that CTCs are capable of co-expressing both epithelial and mesenchymal antigens. It also seems that mesenchymal characteristics facilitate the early stages of metastasis while epithelial characteristics may be needed for the later stages of colonization and for tumor progression.

Factors Regulating EMT and CSC Properties

An EMT can be induced by several alternative signaling pathways, including TGF-beta, Wnt, Notch, and the signaling activated by Hedgehog. In addition, certain developmental transcription factors, specifically Snail1, Slug, SIP1, E12/E47, Zeb1/2, Goosecoid, FOXC2, and Twist, can induce this transition. The expression of some of these transcription factors can be induced during tumor progression and is associated with resistance to apoptosis [38, 75]. The main epigenetic events which play a role in the initiation and maintenance of epigenetic repression or derepression of target genes are DNA methylation, histone modification, nucleosome remodeling, and noncoding RNAs [76, 77]. During EMT and MET the expression of E-cadherin (CDH1), that is one of the main EMT markers, is regulated by multiple mechanism including epigenetic modifications [78, 79]. Furthermore, transcription factors that induce EMT (EMT-TFs), particularly Snail, ZEB, and Twist families, collaborate with a variety of these epigenetic modifiers, including DNA methyltransferases, histone deacetylases, and histone methyltransferase and demethylase, in the transcriptional regulation of CDH1 (reviewed by Lee and Kong [80]). Several studies suggest a crucial role for histone-modifying enzymes in the epigenetic regulation of EMT-TF gene expression [81, 82], supporting the key roles of epigenetic alteration in the regulation of EMT-related factors, including EMT-TFs and EMT markers (reviewed by Lee and Kong [80]).

Recent studies suggested that c-Myc amplification is associated with poor prognosis in various types of cancer, and c-Myc is a common transcription factor for the induction of Snail, ZEB1, and ZEB2 expression [81, 82]. Especially, the c-Myc transcription factor is critical for switching between transcriptional active and repressive components in the epigenetic regulation of EMT-TFs [80]. Because EMT-TFs are closely involved in CSC-associated resistance to an anticancer therapy, targeting EMT-TFs using an epigenetic agent might improve the efficacy of conventional cancer therapy [80].

CTC as a Traveling Diagnostic and Target for Metastasis

Circulating tumor cells represent a unique biomarker, as they are true genuine tumor cells and an integrative part of cancer disease and tumor burden [83]. Moreover, they play a crucial role in tumor dissemination and progression. Even though the presence of CTCs in the peripheral blood was first reported more than 140 years ago [84], only recently advances in molecular biology methods have enabled their reproducible identification and better characterization. The prospect of collecting sequential blood samples for real-time monitoring of systemic therapy efficacy has opened a new avenue for the development of surrogate biomarkers to improve clinical management. Furthermore, a comprehensive molecular characterization of CTCs should provide important insight into the biology of metastasis.

CTCs are extremely rare cells surrounded by billions of blood cells and this represents the main challenge for detection methods to identify and distinguish these cells from normal hematopoietic cells and normal epithelial cells, as well. Several strategies are utilized to achieve this goal including physical and morphologic characteristics like tumor cell weight and size, and/or expression of specific markers (reviewed by [85]). Numerous detection methods are used for the detection of CTCs; however, only part of them demonstrated clinical validity. Taking into account differences in detection methods and markers utilized for CTC definition, various subpopulations of CTCs can be detected that do not necessarily overlap. All data regarding CTCs, including clinical value and expression of therapeutic targets on CTCs for example HER2, hormone receptors, and/or factors related to CTC biology (stem cell markers), should be interpreted within the context of the detection method used [21]. Prognostic value of CTCs was demonstrated by numerous trials for metastatic as well as primary breast cancer using different detection methods [83, 86–89]. However, the CellSearch system (Veridex Corporation, Warren, NJ, USA) is the only FDA-approved system for the detection of CTCs and it has produced the most robust clinical data with reproducible results across different laboratories. The majority of trials used methods that applied a pre-enrichment step using epithelial antigens, such as EpCAM, and/or definition of CTCs as epithelial cells. The consequence may be the underestimation of CTCs with a complete EMT phenotype [53]. However, these cells have been shown to have cancer stem cell properties and to have resistance to chemotherapy and radiotherapy [12].

At present, we have limited data regarding the impact of treatment on detection of CTCs. Phenotypic and genotypic characterization of CTCs could lead to the identification of therapeutic targets on CTCs (for example hormone receptors, HER2 expression, and EGFR expression) [90], and could represent tumor biopsy in "real time." Several groups showed frequent discordance between the HER2 status of tumor primary and CTCs, and case reports showed clinical utility for the use of trastuzumab-based therapy based on the HER2 status of CTCs (reviewed by Mego and Reuben [91]). Similarly, the hormonal status of CTCs could be different from that of the primary tumor, which could lead to an increase of the number of patients suitable for endocrine therapy, but could also explain why endocrine therapy fails in a subset of hormone receptor-positive patients [73]. Several ongoing clinical trials are aimed at determining the predictive value of CTCs in the treatment decision-making process based on CTC count and/or the presence of a therapeutic target on CTCs.

References

1. DeSantis CE, Fedewa SA, Goding Sauer A, Kramer JL, Smith RA, Jemal A (2016) Breast cancer statistics, 2015: convergence of incidence rates between black and white women. CA Cancer J Clin 66(1):31–42
2. Greenberg PA et al (1996) Long-term follow-up of patients with complete remission following combination chemotherapy for metastatic breast cancer. J Clin Oncol 14:2197–2205
3. Gianni L et al (2005) Gene expression profiles in paraffin-embedded core biopsy tissue predict response to chemotherapy in women with locally advanced breast cancer. J Clin Oncol 23:7265–7277
4. Perou CM et al (2000) Molecular portraits of human breast tumours. Nature 406:747–752
5. Pusztai L et al (2003) Gene expression profiles obtained from fine-needle aspirations of breast cancer reliably identify routine prognostic markers and reveal large-scale molecular differences between estrogen-negative and estrogen-positive tumors. Clin Cancer Res 9:2406–2415
6. Kakarala M, Wicha MS (2008) Implications of the cancer stem-cell hypothesis for breast cancer prevention and therapy. J Clin Oncol 26(17):2813–2820. Review
7. Ishikawa F et al (2007) Chemotherapy-resistant human AML stem cells home to and engraft within the bone-marrow endosteal region. Nat Biotechnol 25:1315–1321

8. Li X et al (2008) Intrinsic resistance of tumorigenic breast cancer cells to chemotherapy. J Natl Cancer Inst 100:672–679
9. Liu G et al (2006) Analysis of gene expression and chemoresistance of CD133+ cancer stem cells in glioblastoma. Mol Cancer 5:67
10. Dass K, Ahmad A, Azmi AS, Sarkar SH, Sarkar FH (2008) Evolving role of uPA/uPAR system in human cancers. Cancer Treat Rev 34(2):122–136
11. Thiery JP, Acloque H, Huang RY, Nieto MA (2009) Epithelial-mesenchymal transitions in development and disease. Cell 139(5):871–890
12. Mani SA, Guo W, Liao MJ, Eaton EN, Ayyanan A, Zhou AY, Brooks M, Reinhard F, Zhang CC, Shipitsin M, Campbell LL, Polyak K, Brisken C, Yang J, Weinberg RA (2008) The epithelial-mesenchymal transition generates cells with properties of stem cells. Cell 133(4):704–715
13. Friedl P, Wolf K (2010) Plasticity of cell migration: a multiscale tuning model. J Cell Biol 188:11–19
14. Thiery JP (2003) Epithelial-mesenchymal transitions in development and pathologies. Curr Opin Cell Biol 15:740–746
15. Yilmaz M, Christofori G (2010) Mechanisms of motility in metastasizing cells. Mol Cancer Res 8:629–642
16. Cierna Z, Mego M, Janega P, Karaba M, Minarik G, Benca J, Sedláčková T, Cingelova S, Gronesova P, Manasova D, Pindak D, Sufliarsky J, Danihel L, Reuben JM, Mardiak J (2014) Matrix metalloproteinase 1 and circulating tumor cells in early breast cancer. BMC Cancer 14:472
17. Lozano E, Betson M, Braga VM (2003) Tumor progression: small GTPases and loss of cell-cell adhesion. Bioessays 25:452–463
18. Fidler IJ (1970) Metastasis: guantitative analysis of distribution and fate of tumor embolilabeled with 125 I-5-iodo-2'-deoxyuridine. J Natl Cancer Inst 45:773–782
19. Mego M, Gao H, Cohen EN, Anfossi S, Giordano A, Sanda T, Fouad TM, De Giorgi U, Giuliano M, Woodward WA, Alvarez RH, Valero V, Ueno NT, Hortobagyi GN, Cristofanilli M, Reuben JM (2016) Circulating tumor cells (CTC) are associated with defects in adaptive immunity in patients with inflammatory breast cancer. J Cancer 7(9):1095–1104. doi: 10.7150/jca.13098. eCollection_2016. PubMed PMID: 27326253; PubMed Central PMCID: PMC4911877
20. Mego M, Gao H, Cohen EN, Anfossi S, Giordano A, Tin S, Fouad TM, De Giorgi U, Giuliano M, Woodward WA, Alvarez RH, Valero V, Ueno NT, Hortobagyi GN, Cristofanilli M, Reuben JM (2016) Circulating tumor cells (CTCs) are associated with abnormalities in peripheral blood dendritic cells in patients with inflammatory breast cancer. Oncotarget. doi:10.18632/oncotarget.10290. [Epub ahead of print] PubMed PMID: 27374101
21. Mego M, Mani SA, Cristofanilli M (2010) Molecular mechanisms of metastasis in breast cancer—clinical applications. Nat Rev Clin Oncol 7(12):693–701
22. Hanahan D, Weinberg RA (2011) Hallmarks of cancer: the next generation. Cell 144:646–674
23. Stroka KM, Konstantopoulos K (2014) Physical biology in cancer. 4. Physical cues guide tumor cell adhesion and migration. Am J Phys Cell Physiol 306(2):C98–C109
24. Hollier BG, Evans K, Mani SA (2009) The epithelial-to-mesenchymal transition and cancer stem cells: a coalition against cancer therapies. J Mammary Gland Biol Neoplasia 14:29–43
25. Joyce JA, Pollard JW (2009) Microenvironmental regulation of metastasis. Nat Rev Cancer 9:239–252
26. Karnoub AE et al (2007) Mesenchymal stem cells within tumour stroma promote breast cancer metastasis. Nature 449:557–563
27. Orimo A et al (2005) Stromal fibroblasts present in invasive human breast carcinomas promote tumor growth and angiogenesis through elevated SDF-1/CXCL12 secretion. Cell 121: 335–348
28. Cohen EN, Gao H, Anfossi S, Mego M, Reddy NG, Debeb B, Giordano A, Tin S, Wu Q, Garza RJ, Cristofanilli M, Mani SA, Croix DA, Ueno NT, Woodward WA, Luthra R, Krishnamurthy

S, Reuben JM (2015) Inflammation mediated metastasis: immune induced epithelial-to-mesenchymal transition in inflammatory breast cancer cells. PLoS One 10:e0132710

29. Mego M, Cholujova D, Minarik G, Sedlackova T, Gronesova P, Karaba M, Benca J, Cingelova S, Cierna Z, Manasova D, Pindak D, Sufliarsky J, Cristofanilli M, Reuben JM, Mardiak J (2016) CXCR4-SDF-1 interaction potentially mediates trafficking of circulating tumor cells in primary breast cancer. BMC Cancer 16:127

30. Sarvaiya PJ, Guo D, Ulasov I, Gabikian P, Lesniak MS (2013) Chemokines in tumor progression and metastasis. Oncotarget 4:2171–2185

31. Smolkova B, Mego M, Horvathova Kajabova V, Cierna Z, Danihel L, Sedlackova T, Minarik G, Zmetakova I, Krivulcik T, Gronesova P, Karaba M, Benca J, Pindak D, Mardiak J, Reuben JM, Fridrichova I (2016) Expression of SOCS1 and CXCL12 proteins in primary breast cancer are associated with presence of circulating tumor cells in peripheral blood. Transl Oncol 9(3):184–190

32. Kaplan RN et al (2005) VEGFR1-positive haematopoietic bone marrow progenitors initiate the pre-metastatic niche. Nature 438:820–827

33. Psaila B, Lyden D (2009) The metastatic niche: adapting the foreign soil. Nat Rev Cancer 9:285–293

34. Al-Hajj M, Wicha MS, Benito-Hernandez A, Morrison SJ, Clarke MF (2003) Prospective identification of tumorigenic breast cancer cells. Proc Natl Acad Sci U S A 100(7):3983–3988

35. Ginestier C, Hur MH, Charafe-Jauffret E, Monville F, Dutcher J, Brown M, Jacquemier J, Viens P, Kleer CG, Liu S, Schott A, Hayes D, Birnbaum D, Wicha MS, Dontu G (2007) ALDH1 is a marker of normal and malignant human mammary stem cells and a predictor of poor clinical outcome. Cell Stem Cell 1(5):555–567

36. Fidler IJ (2003) The pathogenesis of cancer metastasis: the 'seed and soil' hypothesis revisited. Nat Rev Cancer 3(6):453–458

37. Mani SA, Yang J, Brooks M, Schwaninger G, Zhou A, Miura N, Kutok JL, Hartwell K, Richardson AL, Weinberg RA (2007) Mesenchyme Forkhead 1 (FOXC2) plays a key role in metastasis and is associated with aggressive basal-like breast cancers. Proc Natl Acad Sci U S A 104(24):10069–10074

38. Yang J, Weinberg RA (2008) Epithelial-mesenchymal transition: at the crossroads of development and tumor metastasis. Developmental Cell 14:818–829

39. Jolly MK, Boareto M, Huang B, Jia D, Lu M, Ben-Jacob E, Onuchic JN, Levine H (2015) Implications of the hybrid epithelial/mesenchymal phenotype in metastasis. Front Oncol 5:155. doi: 10.3389/fonc.2015.00155. eCollection 2015. Review. PubMed PMID: 26258068; PubMed Central PMCID: PMC4507461

40. Jolly MK, Jia D, Boareto M, Mani SA, Pienta KJ, Ben-Jacob E, Levine H (2015) Coupling the modules of EMT and stemness: A tunable 'stemness window' model. Oncotarget 6(28):25161–25174. doi: 10.18632/oncotarget.4629. PubMed PMID: 26317796; PubMed Central PMCID: PMC4694822

41. Jolly MK, Tripathi SC, Jia D, Mooney SM, Celiktas M, Hanash SM, Mani SA, Pienta KJ, Ben-Jacob E, Levine H (2016) Stability of the hybrid epithelial/mesenchymal phenotype. Oncotarget 7(19):27067–27084. doi: 10.18632/oncotarget.8166. PubMed PMID: 27008704

42. Hüsemann Y et al (2008) Systemic spread is an early step in breast cancer. Cancer Cell 13:58–68

43. Stoecklein NH et al (2008) Direct genetic analysis of single disseminated cancer cells for prediction of outcome and therapy selection in esophageal cancer. Cancer Cell 13:441–453

44. Weckermann D et al (2009) Perioperative activation of disseminated tumor cells in bone marrow of patients with prostate cancer. J Clin Oncol 27:1549–1556

45. Baccelli I, Schneeweiss A, Riethdorf S, Stenzinger A, Schillert A, Vogel V et al (2013) Identification of a population of blood circulating tumor cells from breast cancer patients that initiates metastasis in a xenograft assay. Nat Biotechnol 31:539–544

46. Kim MY et al (2009) Tumor self-seeding by circulating cancer cells. Cell 139:1315–1326

47. Norton L (2008) Cancer stem cells, self-seeding, and decremented exponential growth: theoretical and clinical implications. Breast Dis 29:27–36
48. Chaffer CL et al (2006) Mesenchymal-to-epithelial transition facilitates bladder cancer metastasis: role of fibroblast growth factor receptor-2. Cancer Res 66:11271–11278
49. Tsuji T et al (2008) Epithelial-mesenchymal transition induced by growth suppressor p12CDK2-AP1promotes tumor cell local invasion but suppresses distant colony growth. Cancer Res 68:10377–10386
50. Tarin D (2007) New insights into the pathogenesis of breast cancer metastasis. Breast Dis 26:13–25
51. Giordano A, Gao H, Anfossi S et al (2012) Epithelial-mesenchymal transition and stem cell markers in patients with HER2-positive metastatic breast cancer. Mol Cancer Ther 11:2526–2534
52. Kasimir-Bauer S, Hoffmann O, Wallwiener D, Kimmig R, Fehm T (2012) Expression of stem cell and epithelial-mesenchymal transition markers in primary breast cancer patients with circulating tumor cells. Breast Cancer Res 14:R15
53. Mego M, Mani SA, Lee BN, Li C, Evans KW, Cohen EN, Gao H, Jackson SA, GiordanoA HGN, Cristofanilli M, Lucci A, Reuben JM (2012) Expression of epithelial-mesenchymal transition-inducing transcription factors in primary breast cancer:The effect of neoadjuvant therapy. Int J Cancer 130:808–816
54. Yu M, Bardia A, Wittner BS, Stott SL, Smas ME, Ting DT, Isakoff SJ, Ciciliano JC, Wells MN, Shah AM, Concannon KF, Donaldson MC, Sequist LV, Brachtel E, Sgroi D, Baselga J, Ramaswamy S, Toner M, Haber DA, Maheswaran S (2013) Circulating breast tumor cells exhibit dynamic changes in epithelial and mesenchymal composition. Science 339:580–584
55. Bonnomet A et al (2010) Epithelial-to-mesenchymal transitions and circulating tumor cells. J Mammary Gland Biol Neoplasia 15:261–273
56. Ota I, Li XY, Hu Y, Weiss SJ (2009) Induction ofa MT1-MMP and MT2-MMP-dependent basement membrane transmigration program in cancer cells by Snail1. Proc Natl Acad Sci U S A 106:20318–20323
57. Kudo-Saito C, Shirako H, Takeuchi T, Kawakami Y (2009) Cancer metastasis is accelerated through immunosuppression during Snail-induced EMT of cancer cells. Cancer Cell 15:195–206
58. Peinado H et al (2004) Snail and E47 repressors of E-cadherin induce distinct invasive and angiogenic properties in vivo. J Cell Sci 117:2827–2839
59. Shih JY et al (2005) Transcription repressor slug promotes carcinoma invasion and predicts outcome of patients with lung adenocarcinoma. Clin Cancer Res 11:8070–8078
60. Labelle M et al (2008) Vascular endothelial cadherin promotes breast cancer progression via transforming growth factor beta signaling. Cancer Res 68:1388–1397
61. Qi J, Chen N, Wang J, Siu CH (2005) Transendothelial migration of melanoma cells involves N-cadherin-mediated adhesion and activation of the beta-catenin signaling pathway. Mol Biol Cell 16:4386–4397
62. Milsom C, Anderson GM, Weitz JI, Rak J (2007) Elevated tissue factor procoagulant activity in CD133-positive cancer cells. J Thromb Haemost 5:2550–2552
63. Yang J et al (2004) Twist, a master regulator of morphogenesis, plays an essential role in tumor metastasis. Cell 117:927–939
64. Tsai JH, Donaher JL, Murphy DA, Chau S, Yang J (2012) Spatiotemporal regulation of epithelial-mesenchymal transition is essential for squamous cell carcinoma metastasis. Cancer Cell 22(6):725–36. doi: 10.1016/j.ccr.2012.09.022. Epub 2012 Nov 29. PubMed PMID: 23201165; PubMed Central PMCID: PMC3522773
65. Tsuji T, Ibaragi S, Hu GF (2009) Epithelial mesenchymal transition and cell cooperativity in metastasis. Cancer Res 69:7135–7139
66. Mego M, Cierna Z, Janega P, Karaba M, Minarik G, Benca J, Sedláčková T, Sieberova G, Gronesova P, Manasova D, Pindak D, Sufliarsky J, Danihel L, Reuben JM, Mardiak J (2015) Relationship between circulating tumor cells and epithelial to mesenchymal transition in early breast cancer. BMC Cancer 15:533. doi: 10.1186/s12885-015-1548-7. PubMed PMID: 26194471; PubMed Central PMCID: PMC4509773

67. Soini Y, Tuhkanen H, Sironen R, Virtanen I, Kataja V, Auvinen P, Mannermaa A, Kosma VM (2011) Transcription factors zeb1, twist and snai1 in breast carcinoma. BMC Cancer 11:73

68. Aktas B et al (2009) Stem cell and epithelial mesenchymal transition markers are frequently overexpressed in circulating tumor cells of metastatic breast cancer patients. Breast Cancer Res 11:R46

69. Fehm T et al (2007) Determination of HER2 status using both serum HER2 levels and circulating tumor cells in patients with recurrent breast cancer whose primary tumor was HER2 negative or of unknown HER2 status. Breast Cancer Res 9:R74

70. Kallergi G et al (2009) Hypoxia-inducible factor-1alpha and vascular endothelial growth factor expression in circulating tumor cells of breast cancer patients. Breast Cancer Res 11:R84

71. Kallergi G et al (2008) Phosphorylated EGFR and PI3K/Akt signaling kinases are expressed in circulating tumor cells of breast cancer patients. Breast Cancer Res 10:R80

72. Pestrin M et al (2009) Correlation of HER2 status between primary tumors and corresponding circulating tumor cells in advanced breast cancer patients. Breast Cancer Res Treat 118:523–530

73. Fehm T et al (2009) Detection and characterization of circulating tumor cells in blood of primary breast cancer patients by RT-PCR and comparison to status of bone marrow disseminated cells. Breast Cancer Res 11:R59

74. Reuben JM et al (2010) Circulating tumor cells and biomarkers: implications for personalized targeted treatments for metastatic breast cancer. Breast J 16:327–330

75. De Wever O, Pauwels P, De Craene B, Sabbah M, Emami S, Redeuilh G, Gespach C, Bracke M, Berx G (2008) Molecular and pathological signatures of epithelial-mesenchymal transitions at the cancer invasion front. Histochem Cell Biol 130(3):481–494

76. Dawson MA, Kouzarides T (2012) Cancer epigenetics: from mechanism to therapy. Cell 150(1):12–27

77. Jones PA, Baylin SB (2007) The epigenomics of cancer. Cell 128(4):683–692

78. Bedi U, Mishra VK, Wasilewski D, Scheel C, Johnsen SA (2014) Epigenetic plasticity: a central regulator of epithelial-to-mesenchymal transition in cancer. Oncotarget 5(8):2016–2029

79. De Craene B, Berx G (2013) Regulatory networks defining EMT during cancer initiation and progression. Nat Rev Cancer 13(2):97–110

80. Lee JY, Kong G (2016) Roles and epigenetic regulation of epithelial-mesenchymal transition and its transcription factors in cancer initiation and progression. Cell Mol Life Sci. 73(24):4643–4660

81. Cho MH, Park JH, Choi HJ, Park MK, Won HY, Park YJ, Lee CH, Oh SH, Song YS, Kim HS, Oh YH, Lee JY, Kong G (2015) DOT1L cooperates with the c-Myc-p300 complex to epigenetically derepress CDH1 transcription factors in breast cancer progression. Nat Commun 6:7821

82. Choi HJ, Park JH, Park M, Won HY, Joo HS, Lee CH, Lee JY, Kong G (2015) UTX inhibits EMT-induced breast CSC properties by epigenetic repression of EMT genes in cooperation with LSD1 and HDAC1. EMBO Rep 16(10):1288–1298

83. Cristofanilli M, Budd GT, Ellis MJ, Stopeck A, Matera J, Miller MC, Reuben JM, Doyle GV, Allard WJ, Terstappen LW, Hayes DF (2004) Circulating tumor cells, disease progression, and survival in metastatic breast cancer. N Engl J Med 351:781–791

84. Ashworth TR (1869) A case of cancer in which cells similar to those in the tumours were seen in the blood after death. Aust Med J 14:146–149

85. Alix-Panabières C, Pantel K (2014) Challenges in circulating tumour cell research. Nat Rev Cancer 14(9):623–631. doi:10.1038/nrc3820. Epub 2014 Jul 31. PubMed PMID: 25154812

86. Bidard FC, Peeters DJ, Fehm T, Nolé F, Gisbert-Criado R, Mavroudis D et al (2014) Clinical validity of circulating tumor cells in patients with metastatic breast cancer: a pooled analysis of individual patient data. Lancet Oncol 15:406–414

87. Lucci A, Hall CS, Lodhi AK, Bhattacharyya A, Anderson AE, Xiao L et al (2012) Circulating tumour cells in non-metastatic breast cancer: a prospective study. Lancet Oncol 13:688–695

88. Zhang L, Riethdorf S, Wu G, Wang T, Yang K, Peng G et al (2012) Metaanalysis of the prognostic value of circulating tumor cells in breast cancer. Clin Cancer Res 18:5701–5710

89. Zhao S, Liu Y, Zhang Q, Li H, Zhang M, Ma W et al (2011) The prognostic role of circulating tumor cells (CTCs) detected by RTPCR in breast cancer: ameta-analysis of published literature. Breast Cancer Res Treat 130:809–816
90. Payne RE et al (2009) Measurements of EGFR expression on circulating tumor cells are reproducible over time in metastatic breast cancer patients. Pharmacogenomics 10:51–57
91. Mego M, Reuben JM (2014) Prognostic and predictive role of circulating tumor cells in breast cancer. Curr Breast Cancer Rep 6(4):251–259

Chapter 5
Detecting and Monitoring Circulating Stromal Cells from Solid Tumors Using Blood-Based Biopsies in the Twenty-First Century: Have Circulating Stromal Cells Come of Age?

Daniel L. Adams and Massimo Cristofanilli

Abstract Recent advancements in profiling genomic and proteomic aberrations of circulating tumor cells (CTCs) have provided a greater understanding of the underlying biology of tumor dissemination and subsequent metastases. Unfortunately, cancer is a complex disease with cancer growth, progression, and spread all intricately dependent not only on cancer cells, but also on a variety of nonmalignant cell types that make up the cancer environment. The concept of a "liquid biopsy," which has recently gained great traction in the field of cancer research, revolves around analyzing the proteomic and genomic characteristics of CTCs and circulating tumor debris (i.e., circulating tumor DNA, tumor exosomes). However, a key concern of this single focus is the loss of vital information provided by nonmalignant cancer-associated cells, i.e., circulating stromal cells and circulating immune cells. Even though non-cancer immune cells are required contributors to the malignant behavior of tumors and are in many cases "abnormal" themselves, why is their study in "liquid biopsies" largely ignored? In this new era of targeted cancer therapies, i.e., immunotherapies, which target tumor cells and stromal cells, diagnostics for personalized treatment requires the ability to effectively account for both pro-cancerous nonmalignant cells and malignant cells. Given that blood harbors several circulating tumor-derived cells, representing a circulating metastatic niche, we must reevaluate what defines a "blood-based biopsy"(BBB) beyond conventional liquid biopsies to include circulating stromal cells as potential diagnostic targets.

Keywords Cancer-associated macrophage-like cells • Cancer-associated endothelial cells • Blood-based biopsy • Circulating stromal cells • Circulating cancer biomarkers

D.L. Adams (✉)
Creatv MicroTech, Inc., Monmouth Junction, NJ 08852, USA
e-mail: dan@creatvmicrotech.com

M. Cristofanilli
Robert H. Lurie Comprehensive Cancer Center, Northwestern University,
Chicago, IL 60611, USA

© Springer International Publishing AG 2017
M. Cristofanilli (ed.), *Liquid Biopsies in Solid Tumors*, Cancer Drug Discovery and Development, DOI 10.1007/978-3-319-50956-3_5

Stromal Cells Are Universal Constituents Found in All Solid Tumors and the Future of Diagnostics

The tumor stroma consists of a variety of cell types found around, and within, all solid tumors at both the primary and disseminated cancer sites (Fig. 5.1). These cells coevolve with tumor cells aiding in the formation of the tumor microenvironment which may be pro-tumorigenic or anti-tumorigenic, depending on the cellular

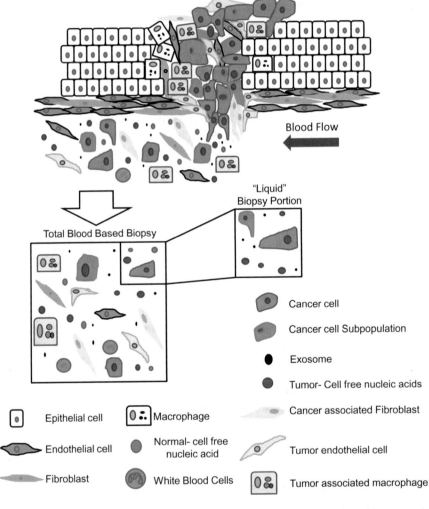

Fig. 5.1 Diagram of a cancer mass with CTCs and CStCs entering the circulation with a comparison of a blood-based biopsy versus a liquid biopsy. In solid tumors a cancerous mass consists of normal epithelial cells, normal resident immune cells, cancerous cell populations, and stromal immune cells. A liquid biopsy will isolate and analyze CTCs, ctDNA, and tumor exosomes. A blood-based biopsy isolates CTCs, other tumor components, and circulating stromal cells which are also found in circulation

response of the host's immune system to the aberrant growth of the cancer [1–6]. Stromal cells can be recruited to the tumor site, or arise from resident cells from the surrounding area, attracted by an inflammatory response to the tumor much like a response to a wound [1–21]. Whether, pro- or anti-tumorigenic, the tumor stroma can make up 90% of a tumor's primary mass which includes connective tissue, capillary vessels, and immune cells, i.e., granulocytes, neutrophils, macrophages, endothelial cells, fibroblasts, adipocytes, lymphocytes, smooth muscle cells, pericytes, and neuroendocrine cells [1, 2, 4, 5, 7, 13, 14, 18, 22]. While a host's immune response to the presence of malignant cells remains a complicated and confusing arena, it also is rapidly becoming a primary topic of research in the oncology field [1–6, 18, 22–28]. Success of immunotargeted therapies, such as immune blockade inhibitor drugs, which specifically alter the host's immune response and therefore the stoma itself, has led to an understanding that stromal cell interaction with tumor cells is the future in studying and treating cancer [1–6, 18, 22–28].

Diagnosis during cancer progression and metastatic spread typically focuses on the tumor cells and their biomarkers, though stromal cells and stromal biomarkers are rapidly moving to the forefront in the study of oncology. We are beginning to understand that stromal cells are key components in the microenvironment of the tumor, playing a prominent role in cancer growth and spread. This has led to the realization that a patient's own lymphatic cellular/immunity response should be analyzed early in a tumor's life cycle and act as a surrogate marker for response during treatment. In the case of pro-tumorigenic stroma, the stromal cells are not themselves inherently tumorigenic, or malignant, but they are intricately involved with tumor initiation, growth, spread, and metastasis of cancer [1–6, 18].

Stromal cell-tumor cell interactions are currently being used to tailor treatments by altering the immune reactions to tumors [1, 3–5, 16, 22–32]. Immune-modulating drugs, for example, affecting the immune checkpoint blockades in stroma, have shown amazing promise in activating a host's immune response to attack tumor cells. These drugs have refocused how oncologists analyze biopsies for diagnosis and the importance of stroma in analyzing drug response. The most recently approved FDA-approved immune-modulator drugs targeting the PD-L1/PD-1 blockade (e.g., nivolumab, atezolizumab, and pembrolizumab) are known to directly affect immune stromal cells. In contrast to classical oncology drug targeting, the receptor PD-1 is not expressed on tumor cells, and while its ligand PD-L1 may at times be present on tumor cells, the ligand is highly expressed on a number of stromal subtypes (i.e., macrophages, endothelial cells, fibroblasts, T-cells, etc.) [22–32]. Further, PD-L1 presence on either stromal cells or tumor cells are indicators of anti-tumorigenic drug response, suggesting that the analysis of all cell types might be necessary to properly assess drug response [22–33]. Further exacerbating the complexity of immune modulators is the fact that the immune reaction to tumors is a dynamic process which changes over time, and with induction of treatment [24, 29–31, 33]. The dynamic nature of immune-modulating drugs has presented issues previously unforeseen in cancer drug utilization: requiring a companion test that accounts for biomarkers present on both tumor cells and nonmalignant stromal cells, but also requiring retesting of patients long after initial treatment and after the tumor has been removed [1, 23, 24, 26–29, 32, 33]. A possible solution to this problem is the "liquid biopsy," whereby blood is used as a surrogate to the actual tumor biopsy, giving oncologists a real-time picture into the current dynamics of a cancer's progression [34–55]. Typically a "liquid biopsy" analyzes circulating tumor cells (CTC), or other tumor cell components found in the blood (i.e., tumor exosomes, tumor cell-free DNA, tumor proteins) (Fig. 5.1) [34–62]). While the current "liquid biopsy" approach fits the criteria of real-time sequential testing of a patient's tumor [46, 47, 51, 63, 64], there remains a need for a more comprehensive blood-based biopsy (BBB) approach. This BBB approach must track the dynamic changes in tumors but also expand past simple tumor analysis to include tumor niche cells, such as stromal inflammatory cells (Fig. 5.1).

Circulating Stromal Cells (CStCs): More Than Just One Needle in a Haystack

The growth and spread of malignant metastatic disease rely on not only tumor-initiating cells (TICs), like CTCs, but also nonmalignant tumor-associated cells (TACs) which are essential in forming the metastatic microenvironment. Recently it has been theorized that a multitude of varying TACs (i.e., cancer-associated fibroblasts [CAFs], tumor endothelial cells [TECs], tumor-associated macrophages [TAMs]) may originate from tumor sites, spread throughout the body, home to metastatic sites, and even reseed the primary tumor site [7–11, 14, 16–19, 56, 64–72]. Interestingly, while it has now become accepted dogma that tumor growth, proliferation, and spread are dependent on multiple TICs and TACs working together in orchestration, very little study has been done on the TAC phenotypes found in patient blood samples [7–11, 14, 16–19, 34, 35, 56, 64–78]. These circulating TACs, recently defined as circulating stromal cells (CStCs), represent subpopulations of the original stromal mass, which we consider as a new and undefined cohort of immune cells. Until recently, high phenotypic variability of TIC and TACs made consistent isolation and cell subtyping problematic. However, recent advances in BBBs including newer molecular/proteomic techniques have made possible more detailed phenotypic subtyping of TICs and TACs [7–11, 14, 16–19, 34, 35, 37, 46–48, 52, 54, 56, 58, 64–82]. Currently, the most commonly studied stromal cells in tumors include monocytes, TAMs, TECs, CAFs, neutrophils, adipocytes, and T cells, though in most literature monocytes, CAFs, and TECs are the primary focus in regard to CStCs.

The primary transitory route for TICs and TACs from primary tumor areas to distal metastatic sites is the circulatory system. For decades, TICs and TACs emanating from the primary tumor mass have been found transiting the circulatory system in patients with solid tumors [7–14, 16, 18–21, 34–36, 39, 40, 52, 54, 64–66, 69–72, 74, 77, 78, 83–86]. The most commonly studied circulating TICs are the CTCs, which are epithelia-derived tumor cells found in the blood of late-stage cancer patients, and a measurable component in metastatic spread. CStCs, i.e., TACs in the circulation, are the nonmalignant immune cells which like CTCs are also found in the blood of cancer patients. CStCs are far less studied than CTCs but have been described as highly prevalent and specific to cancer, i.e., circulating monocytes, endothelial cells, and fibroblasts [7–14, 16, 18–21, 64–66, 69–72, 77, 78, 84–86]. Most of the published researches regarding CStCs use one of the three general isolation methods: white blood cell (WBC) smears after red blood cell (RBC) lysis, flow cytometry, or cell filtration [7–14, 16, 18–21, 64–66, 69–72, 77, 78, 84–87]. RBC lysis/WBC smear is a technique which commonly uses a hypo-osmotic solution to lyse RBCs, but keeps WBCs intact for smearing onto a glass slide [8, 10, 46, 47, 65]. The advantage of RBC lysis/WBC smear is that most non-RBCs will remain intact for analysis after isolation. Disadvantages include (1) the loss of weakened cells (i.e., apoptotic cells) which also lyse during the RBC lysis step, (2) the destruction of large cells which will be mechanically disrupted during the smear step, and (3) analysis of all cells in the smear being time consuming and labor intensive [8, 10, 46, 47, 65]. Flow cytometry uses antibodies to identify the specific cellular proteins expressed by CTCs or CStCs [19, 46, 47, 69, 70]. This technique has been shown to be initially useful in identifying and differentiating CTCs and CStCs from other cells in the circulation [7, 19, 46, 47, 69, 70]. Disadvantages include the following: (1) the loss of weakened cells, as flow cytometry also has an RBC lysis step; (2) the fact that there are presently no universal biomarkers to identify CStCs; (3) some biomarkers which identify CTCs can also be found in CStCs; and (4) flow cells used in flow cytometry cannot process large cells or large cell clusters [7, 8, 12, 19, 34, 42, 46, 47, 52, 54, 56, 65, 66, 69, 70, 72, 77, 78, 88, 89].

Size-based separation of whole-human blood using microfiltration is an attractive technique for blood cell isolation and has been used to successfully isolate CTCs, TECs, and CAFs from the blood of patients with malignant disease (Fig. 5.2) [29, 34, 35, 42, 46, 47, 51, 56, 63, 64, 66, 73–76, 78, 88, 90–102]. Until recently, filtration-based isolation of cells has been accomplished almost exclusively using RBC lysis followed by track-etch filter technique, developed over 60 years ago by Seal et al. [35, 42, 46, 47, 51, 56, 66, 78, 95–98, 100, 101, 103]. These track-etch filters are manufactured with randomly positioned pores and uneven pore diameters, sometimes causing loss of cellular structure and a decrease in cell retention [35]. Recently, advances in microfabrication using photolithography etching have allowed for the reproducible production of high-precision microfilters which preserves cell morphology for cytological analysis using high-resolution microscopy (CellSieve™ microfilters) [29, 34, 35, 59, 63, 64, 73–76, 88, 90–94, 99, 100, 102]. These microfilters have been shown to rapidly and effectively isolate CTCs and CStCs from the whole peripheral blood without RBC lysis or harsh chemical/mechanical manipulation of cells, an issue commonly observed with track-etch technology [35, 45–47, 51, 56, 66, 78, 95, 103, 104]. With the benefits of minimal manipulation, stable isolation, and high-resolution microscopic analysis, CellSieve™ microfilters are able to gently isolate cells for proper identification and different between CTC populations, the newly identified circulating cancer-associated macrophage-like (CAMLs) cells and circulating cancer-associated vascular endo-thelial cells (CAVEs) (Fig. 5.2) [34, 64, 74, 76]. By using a combination of cytologi-

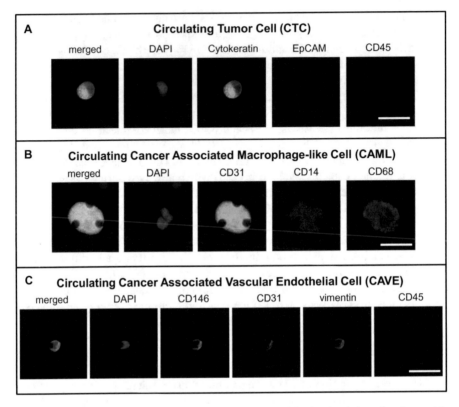

Fig. 5.2 The three most commonly isolated cell types found in the circulation of patients with malignant disease. (**a**) CTCs are rare circulating cells found in patients with late-stage metastatic disease mainly found in breast, prostate, and colon cancer patients. (**b**) CAMLs are a highly prevalent and specific circulating stromal cell subtype, which has been found in over a dozen types of solid cancers. (**c**) CAVEs are also highly specific CStC subtype found in many patients with solid tumors. Scale bar = 30 µm

cal analysis and the commonly used tumor cell biomarkers cytokeratin, epithelial cell adhesion molecule (EpCAM), and CD45, TIC/TACs can be initially identified as CTCs, or CStCs [34, 63, 64, 74–76]. Further, unlike any other BBB approaches, isolated cells on CellSieve™ microfilters can be fully subtyped by restaining with a multitude of CStC subtyping biomarkers (i.e., CD31, CD144, and CD146 for CAVEs and cytokeratin, CD14, and CD45 for CAMLs) [34, 63, 64, 74–76]. As both CAMLs and CAVEs are highly heterogeneous and have also been shown to possess some tumor biomarkers, the combination of multi-biomarker analysis with proper cytological confirmation is paramount in properly analyzing cells in BBBs [34, 63, 64, 66, 74–78]. This issue has been summarized by Adams et al., Cima et al., Magbanua et al., and El-Heliebi et al. describing that CAMLs and CAVEs often present as cytokeratin positive/CD45 negative, and might be confused for CTCs [34, 63, 64, 66, 74–78]. Additionally, as CTCs, CAVE, and CAMLs are all considered rare events which contain similar biomarkers, advancement in BBB approaches will be reliant on the ability to both isolate the various types of TICs and TACs while also properly differentiating between cells with overlapping biomarker phenotypes [34, 63, 64, 66, 74–78].

TAMs and Circulating CAMLs

TAMs, described as one of the most common cellular components in and around tumor masses, have been shown to be recruited from circulating monocytes or derived from resident monocytes [1–6, 11, 13, 15–19, 21, 22, 64, 69]. Often located in tumor stroma, TAMs are prognostic indicators in a number of tumor types, heavily involved in environmental signaling of tumor cells, at times enhancing tumor invasiveness, and at times playing a role in tumor suppression. TAMs have been shown to be involved at every part of a tumor's life cycle, from the invasive front of tumors to partners in cellular intravasation, and even the instigators of microenvironmental niches [1–6, 11, 13, 15–19, 21, 22, 64, 69]. Pro-tumorigenic TAMs regulate and instigate angiogenesis through a number of secreted cytokines and their podosomes can break down extracellular matrices, protruding through endothelial junctions to aid in the spread of CTCs by means of transendothelial migration [2–6, 11, 13, 15–19, 21, 22, 64, 69]. In addition, TAMs are responsible for many tumor debris in blood as they are responsible for phagocytosis and digestion of tumor cells, creating circulating tumor nucleic acids, tumor exosomes, and other exogenous tumor fragments [2–6, 11, 13, 15–19, 21, 22, 58, 60–62, 64, 69]. Further, macrophages are one of the few cells capable of extravasation anywhere in the human body including the lymphatic system, blood, organs, and even across the blood–brain barrier. Add to this the fact that macrophages may express proangiogenic phenotypes (TIE-2) which can recruit other necessary cellular components for tumor growth and spread, it is no wonder that the study of monocytes in cancer is so active.

Circulating CAML analysis has been accomplished almost exclusively by CellSieve™ microfiltration, though the broader tumor-educated monocytes, positive for CD14 and tumor biomarkers, are identified by flow cytometry analysis [11, 19, 63, 64, 69]. While effective at finding CD14+ monocytes, flow cytometry cannot definitively define the cells as stromal derived, nor can it analyze subsets of CD14 low/negative macrophages, found using microfiltration [11, 19, 63, 64, 69]. Recently, Adams et al. have extensively characterized a tumor-specific macrophage-like subtype from patients with malignant disease [63, 64]. Using the previously described low-pressure filtration system and CellSieve™ microfilters, Adams et al. discovered a circulating cancer-associated macrophage-like cell population defined as a CAML [63, 64]. CAMLs were found to be a subtype of CStCs, easily recognized by their aberrant nuclear structures and atypical cell size, usually 30–300 um in diameter. Unlike monocytes or TAMS, which are normal in size (~8 micron) and with a single nucleus, CAMLs were described as a highly differentiated giant polykaryon specific to people with malignant disease, irrespective of cancer subtypes (i.e., breast, prostate, and pancreas cancers) [63, 64]. In the first study of these cells, CAMLs were identified in 83% of patients with stage I/II cancer, and in 92% of all cancer patients. While CD14+ and CD45+ were common in most CAMLs, the cells could be found absent of these markers, making them phenotypically similar to CTCs. Further, some CAMLs contained varying degrees of engulfed cancer epithelial markers, including EpCAM and/or cytokeratin 8, 18, and 19, and prostate-specific membrane antigen (PSMA) in prostate cancer patients [63, 64]. Since their initial discovery, Adams et al. have suggested the utility of CAMLs as a sensitive and specific indicator for presence of malignancy, and have shown that CAMLs are more specific in detecting breast cancer than a breast mammography [63, 64, 86, 94]. Further, Lin et al. have only recently presented that during sequential tracking of CAMLs through multiple rounds of radiation treatment, CAMLs could be found upregulating the immune modulator PD-L1 during induction of radiotherapy [32]. In conjunction, using radiation damage as a marker, Adams et al. were able to show that CAMLs do in fact emanate from the primary tumor mass, proving that CAMLs are in fact a CStC subtype [29, 32].

Tumor Endothelial Cells and the Circulating Cancer-Associated Vascular Endothelial Subtype

Tumor endothelial cells (TECs) are stromal cells required for tumor initiation, survival, and growth. Coevolving with the tumor and forming the vital structures for angiogenesis and neovascularization, TECs are mandatory constituents at all tumor sites, are required for tumor vasculature, aid in priming metastatic niches, and contribute to the molecular instability of tumors [1–6, 8, 16–18, 20, 65, 105]. Dozens of TEC-targeted therapies exist, most notably angiogenesis inhibitors, currently used in conjunction with a variety of anticancer drugs. These drugs deplete the cancer of nutrients and prevent cancer growth by inhibiting formation of cancer vasculature. Endothelial cells found in circulation are known as circulating endothelial cells (CECs) and have been difficult to study due to their vast heterogeneity, aberrant behavior, their presence in malignant disease, presence in nonmalignant disease, and presence in healthy individuals [8, 9, 65, 71, 106]. Currently, there are three common methods for isolating CECs, the CellSearch® CEC assay, RBC lysis/WBC smear, and blood microfiltration [8, 9, 65, 71, 106]. The CellSearch® CEC assay captures a single CEC subtype from blood using antibodies against the endothelial surface marker CD146, and then cells are identified using CD105, and CD45 (to exclude white blood cell contaminates). RBC lysis/WBC smear is effective at isolating and identifying the same endothelial population as the CellSearch® CEC assay, with some increased specificity by using CD146, vWF, and CD45 as CEC biomarkers. Both methods find CECs in various conditions including malignancy and benign diseases (i.e., myocardial infarctions and benign masses) [8, 9, 65, 71, 106]. Interestingly both methods have also shown that an increase in CEC size and clustering is a specific sign of more advanced disease states. Taking advantage of the size specificity observation made by these groups, CellSearch® and RBC/WBC lysis, it has been observed that blood filtration only isolates the specific aberrant subpopulation of TECs, a.k.a. CAVEs, without isolating normal CECs common to other diseases and healthy persons [8–10, 65, 66, 71, 77, 78, 87, 106]. This specificity appears to be partly based on the previous cited observation that normal CECs are small and normal in nature, while CAVEs appear with an unusually large size and the common phenotype of clustering or sheeting [8–10, 65, 66, 71, 77, 78, 87, 106]. Using a filter-based approach, Cima et al. and Magunba et al. profiled CAVEs using the endothelial markers CD31, CD144, and CD146. They suggested that a combination of filtration with CEC markers gives high sensitivity and specificity for isolating only a CAVE subpopulation [66, 77, 78]. However, as these observations were made within the past year, the large-scale clinical utility of CAVE detection and enumeration, as well as their part in the metastatic spread, is currently unknown.

Cancer-Associated Fibroblasts, Neutrophils, and Other Cell Types

Cancer-associated fibroblasts (CAFs) are often the most prevalent nonimmune cells in a tumor's stroma. They are known to modulate cancer cell dissemination and supply the paracrine signaling components during tumor growth and metastatic spread, and facilitate modeling of the tumor [1, 2, 4, 6, 7, 70]. CAFs have been studied for their part in cancer niche formation at metastatic sites and recently it has been shown that their presence in the circulation is an indicator of metastatic spread [1, 2, 4, 6, 7, 70]. While the roles of CAFs are beginning to be elucidated within the tumor stroma, circulating CAFs have been difficult to study. Circulating CAFs transit the circulation, can be found at sites of metastatic spread, and provide a key component of early microenvironmental niche formation. However their isolation and identification have proven difficult. The fundamental issue of fibroblast isolation and detection is their highly diverse, yet embryonic, phenotype. Unlike CTCs, TAMs, and TECs, CAFs have no universal identification markers [1, 2, 4, 6, 7, 70]. Within a solid tumor mass, CAFs are typically defined by their location, spindle shape morphology, and absence of other cell-typing markers. In circulation, cell localization is lost, morphology is nonspecific compared to many WBCs, and absence of markers does not specifically define a cell subtype.

Cancer-associated neutrophils (CANs) are a newly discovered phenomenon and their importance in the stromal mass, and in premetastatic niches, is only now being studied. While neutrophils are the most common WBCs in the bloodstream, the existence of a cancer-associated neutrophil in circulation remains theoretical [67, 84, 107]. Circulating adipose stromal cells have been associated with breast and colon cancer patients. But these cells remain early in the experimental stage and their clinical ramifications are undefined [108]. Cancer-associated platelets have recently been found to cloak tumor cells in circulation, inhibiting natural killer cells from clearing CTCs from the bloodstream. In addition, platelet cloaks appear to enhance metastatic spread, though their source is unknown, and isolation of cloaked CTCs remains experimental [46, 47, 85]. As the field of CStCs is only now being defined and explored, there are likely many other stromal cell types still to be identified and analyzed for their biological and clinical importance.

Presence and Prevalence of CTCs and CStCs in Malignant Disease-Reanalyzing Compiled Data Sets

We have previously published multiple studies on the coexistence of CTCs and CStCs in the circulation of patients with cancer, including breast, prostate, lung, and pancreas [29, 34, 35, 63, 64, 73, 74, 91, 92, 94]. While many types of TICs/TACs have been discovered, to date, our work has focused on three cell types, CTCs, CAMLs, and CAVEs. This is because of their high prevalence in the circulation of cancer patients, their specificity to cancer patients, and the ability to properly subtype these cells using standard biomarkers. Fibroblasts were not included because they have no universal identification markers, so their presence cannot be confirmed.

In the studies used, CTCs were defined by their filamentous cytokeratin, surface EpCAM expression, and absence of CD45 (Fig. 5.2a). Additionally CTCs were identified by both a pleomorphic nucleus and the cytological structure of a pathologically definable tumor cell. These CTCs were proven to be the same population isolated by the CellSearch® CTC Test and therefore highly prognostically valuable. CAMLs were defined by their enlarged multinucleated structure and large atypical cell size (30–300 um in diameter), but were often confirmed with CD45, CD14, or cytokeratin (Fig. 5.2b). In these compiled data sets, CAVEs were defined primarily by their endothelial morphology and positivity for CD31, CD144, and/or CD146 (Fig. 5.2c). In this analysis, we used five previously published clinical data sets, comparing and contrasting the presence and prevalence of CTCs, CAVEs, and CAMLs as they relate to cancer subtype, stage, and specificity (Figs. 5.3 and 5.4). This is the first and only study which specifically compares the three most common TICs/TACs found in the circulation of cancer patients.

Our analysis used published clinical sample sets which included 167 peripheral blood samples of patients with known cancer typing and known stage, run using the standard CellSieve™ assay. The cohort included 42 breast, 35 prostate, 41 pancreas, and 49 lung cancer samples, as well as 34 healthy control samples. The patient sets consisted of 43 stage I, 47 stage II, 31 stage III, and 46 stage IV patients. All patient blood samples were stated as being anonymized peripheral blood samples supplied with written informed consent and according to the local IRB approval at each institution. All healthy control samples were stated as being donated blood with written informed consent and IRB approval. Data points were only used when 7.5 mL whole peripheral blood was initially run using the standard CellSieve™ microfiltration CTC assay. All CTCs and CStCs collected by this size-exclusion technique

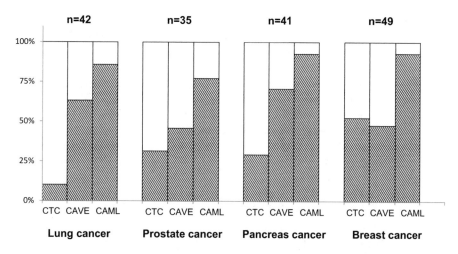

Fig. 5.3 Comparing the prevalence of CAMLs, CAVEs, and CTCs in four different cancer types, $n = 167$. CAMLs are the most prevalent cancer-associated circulating cell found in patients with solid tumors, with 77–93% of cancer patients having at least one CAML per sample of blood. CAVEs are less common than CAMLs but are also found in high prevalence in patients with solid tumor, with 46–71% of patients having at least one CAVE. CTCs are the rarest circulating cells found, most common in breast cancer at 52% and found in only 10% of lung cancer patients

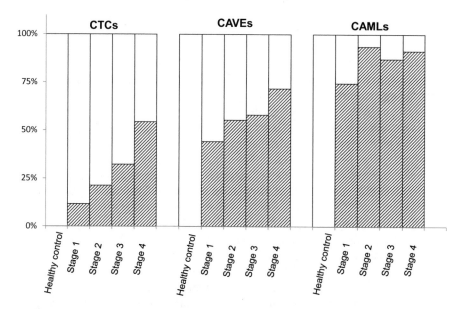

Fig. 5.4 Comparing the prevalence of CAMLS, CAVEs, and CTCs in the four stages of malignant disease with healthy controls ($n = 201$). CAMLs are shown to be a highly specific and sensitive circulating stromal cell subtype found only in patients with malignant disease. CAVEs also appear as specific cellular markers of malignancy, though less common than CAMLs. Unlike CAMLs, CAVEs do appear to numerically correlate with the stage of disease. CTCs are a rarer circulating cell in cancer patients, found in only 12% of stage I patients. However, CTCs are highly correlative to the stage of disease and validated prognostic indicators of patient survival in a variety of malignancies

were fixed, permeabilized, and initially stained with DAPI, antibody cocktail against cytokeratin 8, 18, and 19, EpCAM, CD14, and/or CD45. CTCs and CAMLs were identified as previously described. Samples were then quenched using the quenching, underivatizing, amine stripping, and restaining (QUAS-R); then restained; and reanalyzed for CD31, CD144, and/or CD146. CAVEs were then enumerated and identified as described above [29, 34, 35, 63, 64, 73, 74, 76, 91, 92, 94].

Like many previous studies CTCs, CAMLs, and CAVEs were all shown to be highly specific to malignant disease, with all 34 healthy normal controls being negative for the three cells types: 100% specificity (95% CI 90–100%). At least one TIC/TAC was found in 154 of 167 patient samples, 92% sensitivity (95% CI 97–96%), and only 13 patients were negative for all three cell types. Not surprisingly CStCs were more sensitive than CTCs, with CAMLs the most prevalent cell, found in 145 patient samples, followed by CAVEs found in 96 samples, and CTCs found in 50 patients. Importantly, 76% of patients with CTCs were with late-stage III/IV disease, which matches prior literature concluding that CTCs are specific to late-stage cancers [34, 36, 39, 40, 46, 47, 50–52, 74, 109]. Further, the CTC count is similar to a number of studies using filter technology (~72–83% positivity) as well as the CellSearch® technology, which typically identifies CTCs in late-stage cancers [34, 36, 39, 42, 46, 47, 51, 95, 109]. CAMLs did not seem to have correlation with stage, and were equally common in stages II, III, and IV, but did appear to have a low positivity in stage I disease. This matches the Adams et al. prospective randomized open blinded end-point (PROBE) compliant study on early detection of breast cancer, which concluded that CAMLs were rarer in stage I breast cancer but common in stages II–IV [63]. In contrast to CAMLs, the percent of CAVEs and CTCs were directly related to the stage of disease (Fig. 5.3). In CAVEs and CTCs, stage I disease had the lowest prevalence and stage IV had the highest prevalence. Clearly this data is intriguing and further subtyping analysis is necessary; however in this first comprehensive analysis of CStCs/CTCs this data appears quite promising in utilizing the BBB approach as a diagnostic. In these data sets we compared the utility of a low volume of blood sampling that identified cells in 92% of patients, already an improvement over the use of CTCs alone. Unlike CTCs which are uncommon in early-stage disease, uncommon in lung cancer and uncommon in pancreatic cancer; CStC analysis was applicable to all stages of disease and useful for all tumor subtypes [34, 36, 39–41, 46, 47, 50–52, 74, 109]. Further, while current oncology therapies focus on the expression profiles of the tumor cells themselves, newer immune-modulating therapies are gaining great interest in clinical treatment. These therapies will become more targeted and will be based on expression profiles of tumor cells and tumor-associated cell types, such as TAMS, TECs, and CAFs. Here we supply evidence that an all-in-one BBB can isolate and analyze a multitude of tumor cells and stromal cells all using noninvasive sequential testing of blood samples. In this study, the focus of cell profiling is merely a first step. As this cell-based assaying does not require the plasma, and plasma separation is a step in the CellSieve™ protocol, it is logical to believe that profiling the proteomic and genomic information found in patient plasma may be a next logical step for expanding this assay.

Molecular Abnormalities in Circulation

Mutated DNA is common to all cancer types, found within tumor cells, within stromal cells, and as circulating cell-free DNA (cfDNA) [58, 60, 109–111]. Analyzing tumor DNA from tumor cells has been an area of study for decades, and mutational analysis of tumor DNA is considered standard of care in a number of cancers (i.e., *KRAS/BRAF* mutations in colon cancer, *ALK* rearrangement in *NSCLC* and *HER2* amplification in breast cancer). In liquid biopsies, while enumeration of CTCs as a prognostic indicator is clinically utilized, CTC mutation analysis has been hampered due to the rarity of CTCs and their high mutational heterogeneity. Circulating tumor DNA (ctDNA), as a "liquid biopsy" surrogate for DNA from tumor cells, is a newer concept, but already with an approved FDA test for the *EGFR* mutation subtype (e.g., cobas EGFR mutation test v2). This appears a promising avenue for mutation analysis using blood samples, though sensitivity and specificity of other types of ctDNA remain a concern [60, 109–115]. An immediate option concerning mutational profiling may be in the fact that tumor stromal cells also harbor genomic aberrations, i.e., CAFs, TECs, and TAMs, all known to contain mutations matching the primary tumor mutations [64, 79, 116–122]. While full mutational profiling of CStCs has not been achieved, it is of interest that CAMLs and CAVEs have been described harboring the same genetic aberrations as the primary tumor, but in far higher rates than CTCs and cfDNA [64, 66, 78, 79, 123].

While using blood sampling for mutational analyses is encouraging, the ability to use BBBs as the replacement for tumor cell biopsies must be taken with some deliberation. While CTCs, CStCs, and ctDNA have all been described as containing mutations which can match the primary tumor mass, it must be understood that non-tumor cell genetic instabilities are naturally occurring in all individuals. In stroma, non-tumor genetic instabilities in the TECs, CAFs, and TAMs have been described. Examples of mutations in p53, loss of heterozygosity, and allelic imbalances are found in stromal cells and the role of these mutations in the pathogenesis of the cancer is not fully understood. Likewise, CTCs are a small subpopulation of cells and may not even represent the bulk of the tumor mass. Additionally, clinical trials using mutations in CTCs have not been clinically convincing, and more groups are finding an array of CTC subtypes all with different mutation characteristics [51, 52, 54, 81, 82]. CtDNA while enticing as a simple and general purpose for identifying all DNA from a blood sample has the disadvantage of nonspecificity. CtDNA includes tumor mutations, stromal mutations, and non-deleterious mutations found in all individuals [48, 58, 60, 64, 66, 79, 109–121]. While some groups have shown the ability to identify cancer-driver mutations in cancer patients, these same mutations can be found in aged individuals with no oncogenic conditions [51, 65, 86, 119]. All three cases highlight the difficulty in analyzing aberrant mutations from patient's circulation as stromal cells, nonmalignant cells, and normal cells may harbor mutations unrelated to the cancer pathogenesis.

Immune Checkpoint Therapies and Targeted Therapies, the Future of Cancer Treatment

A new age of immunotherapeutic medicine is arriving for the treatment of oncological diseases. These targeted immunotherapies, and more recently targeted immune checkpoint inhibitor therapies, specifically affect the immunological responses to train them to attack a cancerous growth [23–33]. While these drugs hold great promise in revolutionizing the treatment of cancer, they also are causing a reevaluation of how cancer diagnostics are used. Classically, biomarker analysis in cancer is the primary step in predicting drug response for first-line therapy, as well as subsequent lines of therapy. In cancer biopsy diagnostics, including targeted therapies, a tumor biomarker from an excised tumor is tested in relation to a drug against that specific tumor biomarker (i.e., *EGFR*, *HER-2*, *ALK*). However, when cancer is nonresponsive, recurring, metastatic, or simply difficult to sample, analysis of drug actionable biomarker targets becomes reliant on previous biopsy tissue which can be years old, decades old, or nonexistent [11, 21–23, 40, 42, 81, 83, 101, 102, 111]. Exacerbating the issue is that over time, and intervention, the evolution of the tumor may result in distinctly different cell subpopulations, with proteomic and genomic patterns that are inconsistent with the previous tumor biopsies. This has been documented in the newer immune checkpoint inhibitor therapies which target the host's immune response and the stromal cell interactions with tumor cells, not just the tumor cells themselves. This has created the dilemmas including the following: (1) the classical tumor biopsy may not contain stromal cells, (2) tumor cells in the biopsy may not be the relevant population associated with drug response, and (3) the biopsy may no longer represent the current state of the tumor/stroma [21, 27, 36, 43, 48, 75, 90, 97, 112, 122, 123]. Liquid biopsies have the possibility to overcome some problems by supplying cancer diagnosis in real time. Because extravascular CTCs have a very short lifetime in circulation they may better represent the current biological makeup of the malignancy [46, 109–111]. However, CTCs are a rare event and are largely absent in a number of cancer types (e.g., lung, pancreatic, renal cell cancers) and may disappear completely during interventional therapy. Additionally, tumor cell-specific biomarkers may not be correlated to response with the newer immune checkpoint drug responsiveness [2, 8, 17, 49, 51, 79, 88, 92, 100, 102, 112].

The newest FDA-approved immunotherapies, targeting the PD-L1/PD-1 pathway (e.g., nivolumab, atezolizumab, and pembrolizumab), are potent immune checkpoint inhibitors which have been shown to dramatically regress and stabilize tumors in patients with advanced lung cancer [24–26, 28, 29, 32, 33]. However, nivolumab and pembrolizumab are second-line therapies and highly active only in a very select group of lung cancer patients, ~20% of patients. While numerous attempts have been made to identify a companion diagnostic assay able to predict patient responders/nonresponders, to date the current method using archived biopsies is often inaccurate at differentiating these groups [24–26, 32, 33]. A likely reason for the inaccuracy in these companion tests is that the samples being tested are from localized tumor biopsies, but PD-L/PD-1 expression is not limited to tumor cells.

Surrounding stromal cells and the circulating cells also express PD-L1 and PD-1 [1, 24–26, 28, 31–33, 109]. In addition, nivolumab and pembrolizumab target the receptor PD-1 on T-cells, but current companion diagnostics only test tumor cells for the ligand PD-L1, ignoring PD-L1 expression on stromal cells as well as the actual PD-1-positive cells [1, 24–26, 28, 31–33, 109].

Recently Lin et al. and Adams et al. described that CellSieve™ microfilters can sequentially identify PD-L1-positive cell populations in both CTCs and CStCs from lung cancer patients, tracking PD-L1 expression changes throughout radiotherapy treatment [29, 32]. The study was undertaken knowing that the primary treatment for lung cancer is ionizing radiotherapy which can cause an upregulation of PD-L1 in lung cancer patients [23–29, 31–33]. These studies indicated that response to PD-1/PD-L1 is heavily dependent on treatment and that real-time tracking of PD-L1 expression is a prerequisite for developing future companion diagnostic tests. They suggested that BBBs may represent the current active state of tumors and could track dynamic changes in real time, as treatment progresses. Further, using the CStCs found in the blood of lung cancer patients may be uniquely suitable as a companion test for immune checkpoint therapies.

Total Blood-Based Biopsies: Future Directions

The behavior of human cancer is related not only to the genomic abnormalities of tumor cells but also to the cooperation, or resistance, of the host's immune reaction to the presence of the tumor. In cancer, the inflammatory immune response found within a cancer's stroma provides either a pro- or an anti-tumorigenic microenvironment, aiding tumor progression and spread, or destroying malignancies in its infancy. While most cancer therapies revolve around aberrations within cancer cells, resulting from malignant growth, only recently have therapies begun to address the inhibition of pro-tumorigenic stromal cells and identify clinical usefulness. As cancer treatment becomes more personalized, the array of treatment types is becoming more diverse and directed at not just in the tumor itself, but also the immune reaction to cancer. Despite this recent advancement, stromal cells disseminating from the primary tumor sites remain largely unstudied. Interestingly numerous types of CStCs specific to cancer patients have been described and defined, but they have been largely overlooked. All the necessary cellular and biological components to prime, seed, and grow a metastatic niche can be found within the circulation of cancer patients. From cancer-initiating monocytes to circulating tumor exosomes, the circulation is primed with pro- and anti-tumorigenic biologicals which have yet to be fully studied and analyzed. Despite the potential importance of these circulating cells, no group has evaluated the multitude of tumor-derived cell types, defined an assay which evaluates these CStCs, or developed a more encompassing total blood-based biopsy.

CTCs are considered the seed cells which transit the host's circulatory system colonizing vascular beds and initiating metastatic growths, as well as being the primary center of study in limiting or halting metastatic spread. However, CTCs alone have not, and cannot, explained all of the required steps needed for tumor growth or metastases. Tumor growth, CTC intravasation, migration, extravasation, and growth at distant sites all depend on the interaction of the tumor cell and nonmalignant cellular collaborators. Only with cancer-priming niche cells can a cancer spread to distal sites. Despite the evidence that cancers "bring their own soil" very little has been done studying these cells found in circulation. If true that CAFs, TECs, CAM, and CTCs are all players in the spread of cancer, why are these cells studied as independent and unconnected parts of the tumor puzzle? Aberrant nonmalignant CStCS have been described and defined in many academic studies, though the study of CTCs has always taken center stage and CStCs ignored as an unwelcome contaminants. Interestingly, it has been shown that these aberrant CStCs transit the circulation bound to CTCs, establishing the existence of a detectable and trackable circulating metastatic niche, containing all the necessary components for metastatic initiation[64].

In liquid biopsies, CTC analysis alone has been hampered by the fact that only 30% of patients had any detectable CTCs, and were mostly detected in later stages. Here, we analyzed five previously published studies focusing on the prevalence and specificity of CStC/CTCs in the context of a total BBB in malignant disease. The analysis compiled five clinical studies from 2010–2014 using CellSieve™ microfilters with a low-flow filtration system. By simply identifying CAMLs and CAVEs in the same samples, the sensitivity of cancer-specific cells in circulation increased to 92% (154/167 patients). Importantly, this high sensitivity was matched by 100% specificity when compared to a healthy control population (n=34). The high sensitivity/specificity was achieved using only the standard 7.5 mL of blood sampling; although CellSieve™ microfilters are able to filter more than 7.5 mL, one would presume that increasing the volume input to 15 mL, or even 25 mL, could further improve the sensitivity of this assay [75]. Irregardless of the theoretical possibilities, we suggest that in conjunction with CTCs, CStCs may be useful in tracking changes in treatment, aggressiveness of disease, and identifying possibly drug actionable targets. Together, these studies suggest that BBBs should be used to sequentially and noninvasively isolate both CTCs and CStCs from the patients irregardless of tumor type and tumor stage. As such, accounting for TICs and TACs in the blood may make a BBB uniquely suitable as a companion test for general cancer diagnosis and possibly as a surrogate biomarker for targeted immunotherapies.

A rapid, easy-to-use, reproducible assay to ascertain tumor presence at the earliest possible time point is the goal of most cancer diagnosis assays. However, current cancer diagnosis typically revolves around imaging the tumor to determine spread (using PET, CT, X-ray) or using biomarkers present when the tumor has enlarged to the point of detection (prostate-specific antigen (PSA), carcinoembryonic antigen (CEA), CA15-3, etc.). Likewise, the concept of a liquid biopsy has always focused on the enumeration and profiling of CTCs and tumor components from the peripheral blood of late-stage cancer patients. Using this concept, our understanding in the underlying biology of CTCs has advanced rapidly as genomic and proteomic studies have yielded vast meta-data about CTC subtypes. However, with this plethora of data, CTC research has made no major advancements in curbing or stopping metastasis. If anything, liquid biopsy studies have confirmed that CTCs are as heterogeneous and dynamic as the tumor itself. Further, looking within the circulatory system has shown little promise in the early detection of cancer, as the percentage of CTCs found in patients is too low prior to stage IV disease. Likewise, cfDNA has not yet been able to differentiate malignancy from non-deleterious mutations found in healthy persons, nor can cfDNA be found in early-stage disease. In contrast, the body's natural immune response to cancer is actively reacting to cancerous cells (i.e., NK cells, macrophages, T-cells) long before any liquid biopsy technologies can identify a sizable cancerous growth. It would therefore be logical to look for a lymphatic response as an early indicator of any cancer growth which has become overly aggressive or uncontrollable by the innate immunity response. The ability of stromal immune cells to encapsulate and prevent nodal spread can be found at the earliest of cancer growths, and the most important prognostic factor in many carcinomas. Interestingly, though it is known that stromal cells transit the blood of cancer patients, their enumeration, subtyping, and profiling have been largely ignored. While there have been a few studies evaluating the changes of various WBCs in response to tumor spread, they have met with varying degrees of success [7–9, 11, 14, 16, 17, 19, 21, 29, 63, 64, 66, 67, 71, 72, 78, 84, 92, 94, 107, 108, 116]. In one recent success, a PROBE-compliant study using CAMLs as a marker of malignancy showed extremely high sensitivity and specificity, surpassing even breast mammography in detecting and differentiating benign and malignant conditions [29, 63, 94]. Combined, these studies initially suggest that CStCs can act as a tool in early detection of cancer and as an additional cellular parameter in blood-based diagnostics. By reevaluating prior clinical studies, we suggest that the biological presence of CTCs and CStCs can be used independently from, and in conjunction with, one another to better assess the biological changes in tumor over time, providing companion biomarkers over the entire life of a malignancy. This BBB approach would entail a reanalysis of how we define a liquid biopsy to include all tumor-derived components, from CTCs to ctDNA to CStCs to biologicals not yet discovered.

In conclusion, while liquid biopsies make it possible to interrogate single-tumor cell type in circulation, total blood-based biopsies should make it possible to interrogate the entire tumor's circulating metastatic niche in real time. In particular, the biological values of nonmalignant "atypical" cancer-associated cells are paramount in life cycle of a tumor, in the aggressiveness of malignancies, and in their reaction to immunotargeted therapies. Newer isolation techniques have shown that TACs are common constituents in the circulation of diseased individuals and have raised questions regarding how CTCs are defined. Here we look further, asking the future questions as follows: How are CStCS and CTCs coevolving? How should we evaluate immune cells containing tumor biomarkers? Should we expect that nonmalignant (immune) cells contribute to the malignant behavior of tumors and are themselves "abnormal"? How is the behavior of cancer related to the genomic and proteomic abnormalities of immune cells that cooperate with the malignancy? Since blood appears to harbor several TICs and TACs, representing the circulating metastatic niche, we argue that researchers should investigate these new entities as targets for diagnostics and therapeutic intervention. We suggest that an expansion in blood analysis must be undertaken and that the liquid biopsy be redefined, implying that researchers rethink how they evaluate blood-based diagnostics.

Acknowledgements We would like to thank all of the patients and all of the healthy volunteers who contributed to this study. We also thank Drs. S. Stefansson, D.K. Adams, and C.M. Tang for the help in editing this chapter. This work was supported by the US Army Research Office (ARO) and the Defense Advanced Research Projects Agency (DARPA) (W911NF-14-C0098). The content of the information does not necessarily reflect the position or the policy of the US Government.

References

1. Chen F, Zhuang X, Lin L, Yu P, Wang Y, Shi Y, Hu G, Sun Y (2015) New horizons in tumor microenvironment biology: challenges and opportunities. BMC Med 13:45
2. Dvorak HF (1986) Tumors: wounds that do not heal. N Engl J Med **315**(26):1650–1659
3. Fidler IJ (1970) Metastasis: quantitative analysis of distribution and fate of tumor embolilabeled with 125 I-5-iodo-2'-deoxyuridine. J Natl Cancer Inst **45**(4):773–782
4. Hanahan D, Weinberg RA (2011) Hallmarks of cancer: the next generation. Cell **144**(5): 646–674
5. Tlsty TD, Coussens LM (2006) Tumor stroma and regulation of cancer development. Annu Rev Pathol Mech Dis **1**:119–150
6. Valastyan S, Weinberg RA (2011) Tumor metastasis: molecular insights and evolving paradigms. Cell **147**(2):275–292
7. Ao Z, Shah SH, Machlin LM, Parajuli R, Miller PC, Rawal S, Williams AJ, Cote RJ, Lippman ME, Datar RH (2015) Identification of cancer-associated fibroblasts in circulating blood from patients with metastatic breast cancer. Cancer Res **75**(22):4681–4687
8. Beerepoot L, Mehra N, Vermaat J, Zonnenberg B, Gebbink M, Voest E (2004) Increased levels of viable circulating endothelial cells are an indicator of progressive disease in cancer patients. Ann Oncol **15**(1):139–145
9. Goon PK, Boos CJ, Stonelake PS, Blann AD, GY Lip (2006) Detection and quantification of mature circulating endothelial cells using flow cytometry and immunomagnetic beads: a methodological comparison. Thromb Haemost **96**(1):45
10. Kraan J, Sleijfer S, Foekens JA, Gratama JW (2012) Clinical value of circulating endothelial cell detection in oncology. Drug Discov Today **17**(13–14):710–717
11. Leers MP, Nap M, Herwig R, Delaere K, Nauwelaers F (2008) Circulating PSA-containing macrophages as a possible target for the detection of prostate cancer: a three-color/five-parameter flow cytometric study on peripheral blood samples. Am J Clin Pathol **129**(4): 649–656
12. Masouleh BK, Baraniskin A, Schmiegel W, Schroers R (2010) Quantification of circulating endothelial progenitor cells in human peripheral blood: establishing a reliable flow cytometry protocol. J Immunol Methods **357**(1):38–42
13. Pollard JW (2004) Tumour-educated macrophages promote tumour progression and metastasis. Nat Rev Cancer **4**(1):71–78
14. Schauer IG, Sood AK, Mok S, Liu J (2011) Cancer-associated fibroblasts and their putative role in potentiating the initiation and development of epithelial ovarian cancer. Neoplasia **13**(5):393–405
15. Sone S, Key ME (1986) Antitumor and phagocytic activities of rat alveolar macrophage sub-populations separated on a discontinuous gradient of bovine serum albumin. J Biol Response Mod **5**(6):595–603
16. De Palma M, Mazzieri R, Politi LS, Pucci F, Zonari E, Sitia G, Mazzoleni S, Moi D, Venneri MA, Indraccolo S et al (2008) Tumor-targeted interferon-alpha delivery by Tie2-expressing monocytes inhibits tumor growth and metastasis. Cancer Cell **14**(4):299–311
17. De Palma M, Venneri MA, Galli R, Sergi Sergi L, Politi LS, Sampaolesi M, Naldini L (2005) Tie2 identifies a hematopoietic lineage of proangiogenic monocytes required for tumor vessel formation and a mesenchymal population of pericyte progenitors. Cancer Cell **8**(3):211–226

18. Duda DG, Duyverman AM, Kohno M, Snuderl M, Steller EJ, Fukumura D, Jain RK (2010) Malignant cells facilitate lung metastasis by bringing their own soil. Proc Natl Acad Sci U S A **107**(50):21677–21682
19. Hamm A, Prenen H, Van Delm W, Di Matteo M, Wenes M, Delamarre E, Schmidt T, Weitz J, Sarmiento R, Dezi A (2016) Tumour-educated circulating monocytes are powerful candidate biomarkers for diagnosis and disease follow-up of colorectal cancer. Gut **65**(6):990–1000
20. Harney AS, Arwert EN, Entenberg D, Wang Y, Guo P, Qian B-Z, Oktay MH, Pollard JW, Jones JG, Condeelis JS (2015) Real-time imaging reveals local, transient vascular permeability, and tumor cell intravasation stimulated by TIE2hi macrophage–derived VEGFA. Cancer Discov **5**(9):932–943
21. Szulczewski JM, Inman DR, Entenberg D, Ponik SM, Aguirre-Ghiso J, Castracane J, Condeelis J, Eliceiri KW, Keely PJ (2016) In vivo visualization of stromal macrophages via label-free FLIM-based metabolite imaging. Sci Rep **6**:25086
22. Noy R, Pollard JW (2014) Tumor-associated macrophages: from mechanisms to therapy. Immunity **41**(1):49–61
23. Borghaei H, Paz-Ares L, Horn L, Spigel DR, Steins M, Ready NE, Chow LQ, Vokes EE, Felip E, Holgado E (2015) Nivolumab versus docetaxel in advanced nonsquamous non–small-cell lung cancer. N Engl J Med **373**(17):1627–1639
24. Brahmer J, Reckamp KL, Baas P, Crino L, Eberhardt WE, Poddubskaya E, Antonia S, Pluzanski A, Vokes EE, Holgado E et al (2015) Nivolumab versus docetaxel in advanced squamous-cell non-small-cell lung cancer. N Engl J Med **373**(2):123–135
25. Callahan MK, Ott PA, Odunsi K, Bertolini SV, Pan LS, Venhaus RR, Karakunnel JJ, Hodi FS, Wolchok JD (2014) A phase 1 study to evaluate the safety and tolerability of MEDI4736, an anti-PD-L1 antibody, in combination with tremelimumab in patients with advanced solid tumors. In: ASCO Annual Meeting Proceedings 2014:TPS3120
26. Rizvi NA, Mazières J, Planchard D, Stinchcombe TE, Dy GK, Antonia SJ, Horn L, Lena H, Minenza E, Mennecier B (2015) Activity and safety of nivolumab, an anti-PD-1 immune checkpoint inhibitor, for patients with advanced, refractory squamous non-small-cell lung cancer (CheckMate 063): a phase 2, single-arm trial. Lancet Oncol **16**(3):257–265
27. Rosenberg SA (2014) Decade in review—cancer immunotherapy: Entering the mainstream of cancer treatment. Nat Rev Clin Oncol 11(11):630–632
28. Sundar R, Cho B-C, Brahmer JR, Soo RA (2015) Nivolumab in NSCLC: latest evidence and clinical potential. Therapeutic Adv Med Oncol 7(2):85–96
29. Adams DL, Edelman MJ, Fang P, Jiang W, He J, Xu T, Gao H, Reuben JM, Qiao Y, Hahn S, Lin S (2016) Sequential tracking of PD-L1 expression and RAD50 induction in CTCs and circulating stromal cells of lung cancer patients during treatment with radiotherapy. Cancer Res 76(14 Supplement):4990–4990
30. Demaria S, Golden EB, Formenti SC (2015) Role of local radiation therapy in cancer immunotherapy. JAMA Oncol 1(9):1325–1332
31. Derer A, Deloch L, Rubner Y, Fietkau R, Frey B, Gaipl US (2015) Radio-immunotherapy-induced immunogenic cancer cells as basis for induction of systemic anti-tumor immune responses–pre-clinical evidence and ongoing clinical applications. Front Immunol 6:505
32. Lin SH, He J, Edelman M, Xu T, Gao H, Reuben J, Qiao Y, Liu H, Amstutz P, Hahn S, Adams DL (2015) Sequential assessment of DNA damage response and PD-L1 expression in circulating tumor cells of lung cancer patients during Radiotherapy. J Thorac Oncol:S266–S267
33. Ma W, Gilligan BM, Yuan J, Li T (2016) Current status and perspectives in translational biomarker research for PD-1/PD-L1 immune checkpoint blockade therapy. J Hematol Oncol 9(1):1
34. Adams DL, Stefansson S, Haudenschild C, Martin SS, Charpentier M, Chumsri S, Cristofanilli M, Tang CM, Alpaugh RK (2015) Cytometric characterization of circulating tumor cells captured by microfiltration and their correlation to the cellsearch((R)) CTC test. Cytometry A 87(2):137–144

35. Adams DL, Zhu P, Makarova OV, Martin SS, Charpentier M, Chumsri S, Li S, Amstutz P, Tang CM (2014) The systematic study of circulating tumor cell isolation using lithographic microfilters. RSC Adv 9:4334–4342

36. Allard WJ, Matera J, Miller MC, Repollet M, Connelly MC, Rao C, Tibbe AG, Uhr JW, Terstappen LW (2004) Tumor cells circulate in the peripheral blood of all major carcinomas but not in healthy subjects or patients with nonmalignant diseases. Clin Cancer Res 10(20):6897–6904

37. Cohen SJ, Alpaugh RK, Gross S, O'Hara SM, Smirnov DA, Terstappen LW, Allard WJ, Bilbee M, Cheng JD, Hoffman JP et al (2006) Isolation and characterization of circulating tumor cells in patients with metastatic colorectal cancer. Clin Colorectal Cancer 6(2):125–132

38. Cohen SJ, Punt CJ, Iannotti N, Saidman BH, Sabbath KD, Gabrail NY, Picus J, Morse M, Mitchell E, Miller MC et al (2008) Relationship of circulating tumor cells to tumor response, progression-free survival, and overall survival in patients with metastatic colorectal cancer. J Clin Oncol Off J Am Soc Clin Oncol 26(19):3213–3221

39. Cristofanilli M, Budd GT, Ellis MJ, Stopeck A, Matera J, Miller MC, Reuben JM, Doyle GV, Allard WJ, Terstappen LW et al (2004) Circulating tumor cells, disease progression, and survival in metastatic breast cancer. N Engl J Med 351(8):781–791

40. Danila DC, Fleisher M, Scher HI (2011) Circulating tumor cells as biomarkers in prostate cancer. Clin Cancer Res 17(12):3903–3912

41. de Bono JS, Scher HI, Montgomery RB, Parker C, Miller MC, Tissing H, Doyle GV, Terstappen LW, Pienta KJ, Raghavan D (2008) Circulating tumor cells predict survival benefit from treatment in metastatic castration-resistant prostate cancer. Clin Cancer Res 14(19):6302–6309

42. Farace F, Massard C, Vimond N, Drusch F, Jacques N, Billiot F, Laplanche A, Chauchereau A, Lacroix L, Planchard D et al (2011) A direct comparison of CellSearch and ISET for circulating tumour-cell detection in patients with metastatic carcinomas. Br J Cancer 105(6):847–853

43. Ferreira MM, Ramani VC, Jeffrey SS (2016) Circulating Tumor Cell Technologies. Mol Oncol 10(3):374–394

44. Kagan M, Howard D, Bendele T, Mayes J, Silvia J, Repollet M, Doyle J, Allard J, Tu N, Bui T et al (2002) A sample preparation and analysis system for identification of circulating tumor cells. J Clin Ligand Assay 25(1):104–110

45. Krebs MG, Metcalf RL, Carter L, Brady G, Blackhall FH, Dive C (2014) Molecular analysis of circulating tumour cells [mdash] biology and biomarkers. Nat Rev Clin Oncol 11(3):129–144

46. Lianidou ES, Markou A (2011) Circulating tumor cells in breast cancer: detection systems, molecular characterization, and future challenges. Clin Chem 57(9):1242–1255

47. Lianidou ES, Markou A (2011) Circulating tumor cells as emerging tumor biomarkers in breast cancer. Clin Chem Lab Med 49(10):1579–1590

48. MassardC, OulhenM, Le MoulecS, AugerN, FoulonS, Abou-LovergneA, BilliotF, ValentA, MartyV, LoriotY (2016) Phenotypic and genetic heterogeneity of tumor tissue and circulating tumor cells in patients with metastatic castrationresistant prostate cancer: a report from the PETRUS prospective study. Oncotarget

49. O'Flaherty JD, Gray S, Richard D, Fennell D, O'Leary JJ, Blackhall FH, O'Byrne KJ (2012) Circulating tumour cells, their role in metastasis and their clinical utility in lung cancer. Lung Cancer 76(1):19–25

50. Paoletti C, Muniz MC, Thomas DG, Griffith KA, Kidwell KM, Tokudome N, Brown ME, Aung K, Miller MC, Blossom DL et al (2015) Development of circulating tumor cell-endocrine therapy index in patients with hormone receptor-positive breast cancer. Clin Cancer Res 21(11):2487–2498

51. Paterlini-Brechot P, Benali NL (2007) Circulating tumor cells (CTC) detection: clinical impact and future directions. Cancer Lett 253(2):180–204

52. Punnoose EA, Atwal SK, Spoerke JM, Savage H, Pandita A, Yeh RF, Pirzkall A, Fine BM, Amler LC, Chen DS et al (2010) Molecular biomarker analyses using circulating tumor cells. PLoS One 5(9):e12517

53. Stott SL, Lee RJ, Nagrath S, Yu M, Miyamoto DT, Ulkus L, Inserra EJ, Ulman M, Springer S, Nakamura Z et al (2010) Isolation and characterization of circulating tumor cells from patients with localized and metastatic prostate cancer. Sci Transl Med 2(25):25ra23

54. Yu M, Bardia A, Wittner BS, Stott SL, Smas ME, Ting DT, Isakoff SJ, Ciciliano JC, Wells MN, Shah AM et al (2013) Circulating breast tumor cells exhibit dynamic changes in epithelial and mesenchymal composition. Science 339(6119):580–584

55. Yu M, Stott S, Toner M, Maheswaran S, Haber DA (2011) Circulating tumor cells: approaches to isolation and characterization. J Cell Biol 192(3):373–382

56. Coumans FA, Doggen CJ, Attard G, de Bono JS, Terstappen LW (2010) All circulating EpCAM+CK+CD45- objects predict overall survival in castration-resistant prostate cancer. Ann Oncol 21(9):1851–1857

57. Ginestier C, Hur MH, Charafe-Jauffret E, Monville F, Dutcher J, Brown M, Jacquemier J, Viens P, Kleer CG, Liu S et al (2007) ALDH1 is a marker of normal and malignant human mammary stem cells and a predictor of poor clinical outcome. Cell Stem Cell 1(5):555–567

58. Lanman RB, Mortimer SA, Zill OA, Sebisanovic D, Lopez R, Blau S, Collisson EA, Divers SG, Hoon DS, Kopetz ES (2015) Analytical and clinical validation of a digital sequencing panel for quantitative, highly accurate evaluation of cell-free circulating tumor DNA. PLoS One 10(10):e0140712

59. Stefansson S, Adams DL, Tang C-M (2013) Isolation of Low Abundance Proteins and Cells Using Buoyant Glass Microbubble Chromatography. Chromatogr Res Int 2013:1–6

60. Volik S, Alcaide M, Morin RD, Collins CC (2016) Cell-free DNA (cfDNA): clinical significance and utility in cancer shaped by emerging technologies. Mol Cancer Res 4(10): 898–908

61. Melo SA, Sugimoto H, O'Connell JT, Kato N, Villanueva A, Vidal A, Qiu L, Vitkin E, Perelman LT, Melo CA (2014) Cancer exosomes perform cell-independent microRNA biogenesis and promote tumorigenesis. Cancer cell 26(5):707–721

62. Webber J, Steadman R, Mason MD, Tabi Z, Clayton A (2010) Cancer exosomes trigger fibroblast to myofibroblast differentiation. Cancer Res 70(23):9621–9630

63. Adams DL, Adams DK, Alpaugh RK, Cristofanilli M, Martin SS, Chumsri S, Tang CM, Marks JR (2016) Circulating Cancer-Associated Macrophage-Like Cells Differentiate Malignant Breast Cancer and Benign Breast Conditions. Cancer Epidemiol Biomark Prev 25(7):1037–1042

64. Adams DL, Martin SS, Alpaugh RK, Charpentier M, Tsai S, Bergan RC, Ogden IM, Catalona W, Chumsri S, Tang CM et al (2014) Circulating giant macrophages as a potential biomarker of solid tumors. Proc Natl Acad Sci U S A 111(9):3514–3519

65. Bethel K, Luttgen MS, Damani S, Kolatkar A, Lamy R, Sabouri-Ghomi M, Topol S, Topol EJ, Kuhn P (2014) Fluid phase biopsy for detection and characterization of circulating endothelial cells in myocardial infarction. Phys Biol 11(1):016002

66. Cima I, Kong SL, Sengupta D, Tan IB, Phyo WM, Lee D, Hu M, Iliescu C, Alexander I, Goh WL et al (2016) Tumor-derived circulating endothelial cell clusters in colorectal cancer. Sci Transl Med 8(345):345ra389

67. Coffelt SB, Wellenstein MD, de Visser KE (2016) Neutrophils in cancer: neutral no more. Nat Rev Cancer 16(7):431–446

68. Ishii G, Ito TK, Aoyagi K, Fujimoto H, Chiba H, Hasebe T, Fujii S, Nagai K, Sasaki H, Ochiai A (2007) Presence of human circulating progenitor cells for cancer stromal fibroblasts in the blood of lung cancer patients. Stem Cells 25(6):1469–1477

69. Japink D, Leers MP, Sosef MN, Nap M (2009) CEA in activated macrophages. New diagnostic possibilities for tumor markers in early colorectal cancer. Anticancer Res 29(8): 3245–3251

70. Jones ML, Siddiqui J, Pienta KJ, Getzenberg RH (2013) Circulating fibroblast-like cells in men with metastatic prostate cancer. Prostate 73(2):176–181

71. Rowand JL, Martin G, Doyle GV, Miller MC, Pierce MS, Connelly MC, Rao C, Terstappen LW (2007) Endothelial cells in peripheral blood of healthy subjects and patients with metastatic carcinomas. Cytometry A 71(2):105–113

72. Strijbos M, Gratama J-W, Kraan J, Lamers C, Den Bakker M, Sleijfer S (2008) Circulating endothelial cells in oncology: pitfalls and promises. Br J Cancer 98(11):1731–1735
73. Adams D, Alpaugh RK, Cristofanilli M, Martin S, Chumsri S, Charpentier M, Bergan RC, Ogden IM, Tsai S, Zhu P (2013) Identifying and subtyping circulating tumor cells from breast, prostate, and pancreatic cancer patients based on distinct morphology. Cancer Res 73(8 Supplement):1448–1448
74. Adams DL, Adams DK, Stefansson S, Haudenschild C, Martin SS, Charpentier M, Chumsri S, Cristofanilli M, Tang CM, Alpaugh RK (2016) Mitosis in circulating tumor cells stratifies highly aggressive breast carcinomas. Breast Cancer Res BCR 18(1):44
75. Adams DL, Alpaugh RK, Martin SS, Charpentier M, Chumsri S, Cristofanilli M, Adams DK, Makarova OV, Zhu P, Li S et al (2016) Precision microfilters as an all in one system for multiplex analysis of circulating tumor cells. RSC Adv 6(8):6405–6414
76. Adams DL, Alpaugh RK, Tsai S, Tang CM, Stefansson S (2016) Multi-Phenotypic subtyping of circulating tumor cells using sequential fluorescent quenching and restaining. Sci Rep 6:33488
77. El-Heliebi A, Kroneis T, Zohrer E, Haybaeck J, Fischereder K, Kampel-Kettner K, Zigeuner R, Pock H, Riedl R, Stauber R et al (2013) Are morphological criteria sufficient for the identification of circulating tumor cells in renal cancer? J Transl Med 11:214
78. Magbanua MJ, Pugia M, Lee JS, Jabon M, Wang V, Gubens M, Marfurt K, Pence J, Sidhu H, Uzgiris A et al (2015) A Novel Strategy for Detection and Enumeration of Circulating Rare Cell Populations in Metastatic Cancer Patients Using Automated Microfluidic Filtration and Multiplex Immunoassay. PLoS One 10(10):e0141166
79. Leversha MA, Han J, Asgari Z, Danila DC, Lin O, Gonzalez-Espinoza R, Anand A, Lilja H, Heller G, Fleisher M et al (2009) Fluorescence in situ hybridization analysis of circulating tumor cells in metastatic prostate cancer. Clin Cancer Res 15(6):2091–2097
80. Lohr JG, Adalsteinsson VA, Cibulskis K, Choudhury AD, Rosenberg M, Cruz-Gordillo P, Francis JM, Zhang CZ, Shalek AK, Satija R et al (2014) Whole-exome sequencing of circulating tumor cells provides a window into metastatic prostate cancer. Nat Biotechnol 32(5):479–484
81. Polzer B, Medoro G, Pasch S, Fontana F, Zorzino L, Pestka A, Andergassen U, Meier-Stiegen F, Czyz ZT, Alberter B et al (2014) Molecular profiling of single circulating tumor cells with diagnostic intention. EMBO Mol Med 6(11):1371–1386
82. Powell AA, Talasaz AH, Zhang H, Coram MA, Reddy A, Deng G, Telli ML, Advani RH, Carlson RW, Mollick JA et al (2012) Single cell profiling of circulating tumor cells: transcriptional heterogeneity and diversity from breast cancer cell lines. PLoS One 7(5):e33788
83. Cima I, Wen Yee C, Iliescu FS, Phyo WM, Lim KH, Iliescu C, Tan MH (2013) Label-free isolation of circulating tumor cells in microfluidic devices: Current research and perspectives. Biomicrofluidics 7(1):11810
84. Demers M, Krause DS, Schatzberg D, Martinod K, Voorhees JR, Fuchs TA, Scadden DT, Wagner DD (2012) Cancers predispose neutrophils to release extracellular DNA traps that contribute to cancer-associated thrombosis. Proc Natl Acad Sci 109(32):13076–13081
85. Egan K, Crowley D, Smyth P, O'Toole S, Spillane C, Martin C, Gallagher M, Canney A, Norris L, Conlon N (2011) Platelet adhesion and degranulation induce pro-survival and pro-angiogenic signalling in ovarian cancer cells. PLoS One 6(10):e26125
86. Hume R, West JT, Malmgren RA, Chu EA (1964) Quantitative observations of circulating megakaryocytes in the blood of patients with cancer. N Engl J Med 270(3):111–117
87. Kraan J, Strijbos MH, Sieuwerts AM, Foekens JA, den Bakker MA, Verhoef C, Sleijfer S, Gratama JW (2012) A new approach for rapid and reliable enumeration of circulating endothelial cells in patients. J Thromb Haemost 10(5):931–939
88. Adams DL, Makarova O, Zhu P, Li S, Amstutz P, Tang C (2011) Isolation of circulating tumor cells by size exclusion using lithography fabricated precision microfilters. Proceedings of the 102nd Annual Meeting of the American Association for Cancer Research Cancer Res **71**(8):2369

89. Vona G, Estepa L, Beroud C, Damotte D, Capron F, Nalpas B, Mineur A, Franco D, Lacour B, Pol S et al (2004) Impact of cytomorphological detection of circulating tumor cells in patients with liver cancer. Hepatology 39(3):792–797

90. Adams D, Makarova O, Zu P, (2011) Isolation of circulating tumor cells by size exclusion using lithography fabricated precision microfilters. Proceedings 102nd AACR Meeting 71(8 supplement 2369–2369)

91. Adams D, Martin S, Chumsri S, Charpentier M, Alpaugh R, Cristofanilli M, Tang C, Haudenschild C (2015) Applying a mitotic index to circulating tumor cells and its prognostic significance: A cytological approach to patient **stratification**. J Clin Oncol **33**:11029 ASCO Annual Meeting Proceedings

92. Adams D, Tsai S, Makarova OV, Zhu P, Li S, Amstutz PT, Tang C-M (2013) Low cytokeratin- and low EpCAM-expressing circulating tumor cells in pancreatic cancer. J Clin Oncol **31**:11046 ASCO Annual Meeting Proceedings

93. Adams D, Zhu P, Makarova O, Li S, Amstutz P, Tang C (2012) HER-2 FISH analysis and H & E staining of circulating tumor cells pre-isolated using high porosity precision microfilters. Cancer Res 72(8 Supplement):2395–2395

94. Adams DL, Bergan RC, Martin SS, Chumsri S, Charpentier M, Lapidus RG, Alpaugh RK, Cristofanilli M, Tsai S, Tang C-M (2015) Correlation of cancer-associated macrophage-like cells with systemic therapy and pathological stage in numerous malignancies. J Clin Oncol 2015:11095 ASCO Annual Meeting Proceedings

95. Coumans FA, van Dalum G, Beck M, Terstappen LW (2013) Filter characteristics influencing circulating tumor cell enrichment from whole blood. PLoS One 8(4):e61770

96. Hosokawa M, Hayata T, Fukuda Y, Arakaki A, Yoshino T, Tanaka T, Matsunaga T (2010) Size-selective microcavity array for rapid and efficient detection of circulating tumor cells. Anal Chem 82(15):6629–6635

97. LimLS, HuM, HuangMC, CheongWC, GanAT, LooiXL, LeongSM, Koay ES, Li MH: Microsieve lab-chip device for rapid enumeration and fluorescence in situ hybridization of circulating tumor cells. Lab Chip2012.

98. Lin HK, Zheng S, Williams AJ, Balic M, Groshen S, Scher HI, Fleisher M, Stadler W, Datar RH, Tai YC et al (2010) Portable filter-based microdevice for detection and characterization of circulating tumor cells. Clin Cancer Res 16(20):5011–5018

99. Makarova OV, Adams DL, Divan R, Rosenmann D, Zhu P, Li S, Amstutz P, Tang CM (2016) Polymer microfilters with nanostructured surfaces for the culture of circulating cancer cells. Mater Sci Eng C 66:193–198

100. Stefansson S, Adams DL, Ershler WB, Le H, Ho DH (2016) A cell transportation solution that preserves live circulating tumor cells in patient blood samples. BMC Cancer 16(1):300

101. Zheng S, Lin H, Liu JQ, Balic M, Datar R, Cote RJ, Tai YC (2007) Membrane microfilter device for selective capture, electrolysis and genomic analysis of human circulating tumor cells. J Chromatogr 1162(2):154–161

102. Zhu P, Stanton ML, Castle EP, Joseph RW, Adams DL, Li S, Amstutz P, Tang CM, Ho TH (2016) Detection of tumor-associated cells in cryopreserved peripheral blood mononuclear cell samples for retrospective analysis. J Transl Med 14(1):198

103. Seal SH (1964) A Sieve for the Isolation of Cancer Cells and Other Large Cells from the Blood. Cancer 17:637–642

104. Krebs MG, Hou JM, Sloane R, Lancashire L, Priest L, Nonaka D, Ward TH, Backen A, Clack G, Hughes A et al (2012) Analysis of circulating tumor cells in patients with non-small cell lung cancer using epithelial marker-dependent and -independent approaches. J Thorac Oncol 7(2):306–315

105. Chang YS, di Tomaso E, McDonald DM, Jones R, Jain RK, Munn LL (2000) Mosaic blood vessels in tumors: frequency of cancer cells in contact with flowing blood. Proc Natl Acad Sci U S A 97(26):14608–14613

106. Damani S, Bacconi A, Libiger O, Chourasia AH, Serry R, Gollapudi R, Goldberg R, Rapeport K, Haaser S, Topol S et al (2012) Characterization of circulating endothelial cells in acute myocardial infarction. Sci Transl Med 4(126):126ra133

107. Tuting T, de Visser KE (2016) CANCER. How neutrophils promote metastasis. Science 352(6282):145–146

108. Ghosh S, Hughes D, Parma DL, Ramirez A, Li R (2014) Association of obesity and circulating adipose stromal cells among breast cancer survivors. Mol Biol Rep 41(5):2907–2916

109. Alix-Panabières C, Pantel K (2013) Circulating tumor cells: liquid biopsy of cancer. Clin Chem 59(1):110–118

110. Crowley E, Di Nicolantonio F, Loupakis F, Bardelli A (2013) Liquid biopsy: monitoring cancer-genetics in the blood. Nat Rev Clin Oncol 10(8):472–484

111. Diaz LA, Bardelli A (2014) Liquid biopsies: genotyping circulating tumor DNA. J Clin Oncol 32(6):579–586

112. Genovese G, Kahler AK, Handsaker RE, Lindberg J, Rose SA, Bakhoum SF, Chambert K, Mick E, Neale BM, Fromer M et al (2014) Clonal hematopoiesis and blood-cancer risk inferred from blood DNA sequence. N Engl J Med 371(26):2477–2487

113. Jaiswal S, Fontanillas P, Flannick J, Manning A, Grauman PV, Mar BG, Lindsley RC, Mermel CH, Burtt N, Chavez A et al (2014) Age-related clonal hematopoiesis associated with adverse outcomes. N Engl J Med 371(26):2488–2498

114. Martincorena I, Roshan A, Gerstung M, Ellis P, Van Loo P, McLaren S, Wedge DC, Fullam A, Alexandrov LB, Tubio JM et al (2015) Tumor evolution. High burden and pervasive positive selection of somatic mutations in normal human skin. Science 348(6237):880–886

115. Xie M, Lu C, Wang J, McLellan MD, Johnson KJ, Wendl MC, McMichael JF, Schmidt HK, Yellapantula V, Miller CA et al (2014) Age-related mutations associated with clonal hematopoietic expansion and malignancies. Nat Med 20(12):1472–1478

116. Hida K, Hida Y, Amin DN, Flint AF, Panigrahy D, Morton CC, Klagsbrun M (2004) Tumor-associated endothelial cells with cytogenetic abnormalities. Cancer Res 64(22):8249–8255

117. Hill R, Song Y, Cardiff RD, Van Dyke T (2005) Selective evolution of stromal mesenchyme with p53 loss in response to epithelial tumorigenesis. Cell 123(6):1001–1011

118. Houghton J, Li H, Fan X, Liu Y, Liu JH, Rao VP, Poutahidis T, Taylor CL, Jackson EA, Hewes C et al (2010) Mutations in bone marrow-derived stromal stem cells unmask latent malignancy. Stem Cells Dev 19(8):1153–1166

119. Iguchi Y, Ito YM, Kataoka F, Nomura H, Tanaka H, Chiyoda T, Hashimoto S, Nishimura S, Takano M, Yamagami W et al (2014) Simultaneous analysis of the gene expression profiles of cancer and stromal cells in endometrial cancer. Genes Chromosomes Cancer 53(9):725–737

120. Kinseth MA, Jia Z, Rahmatpanah F, Sawyers A, Sutton M, Wang-Rodriguez J, Mercola D, McGuire KL (2014) Expression differences between African American and Caucasian prostate cancer tissue reveals that stroma is the site of aggressive changes. Int J Cancer 134(1):81–91

121. Patocs A, Zhang L, Xu Y, Weber F, Caldes T, Mutter GL, Platzer P, Eng C (2007) Breast-cancer stromal cells with TP53 mutations and nodal metastases. N Engl J Med 357(25):2543–2551

122. Ricci-Vitiani L, Pallini R, Biffoni M, Todaro M, Invernici G, Cenci T, Maira G, Parati EA, Stassi G, Larocca LM et al (2010) Tumour vascularization via endothelial differentiation of glioblastoma stem-like cells. Nature 468(7325):824–828

123. Pailler E, Auger N, Lindsay CR, Vielh P, Islas-Morris-Hernandez A, Borget I, Ngo-Camus M, Planchard D, Soria JC, Besse B et al (2015) High level of chromosomal instability in circulating tumor cells of ROS1-rearranged non-small-cell lung cancer. Ann Oncol 26(7):1408–1415

Chapter 6
Circulating Free Tumor DNA (ctDNA): The Real-Time Liquid Biopsy

Kelly Kyker-Snowman and Ben Ho Park

Abstract It is now well established that DNA is shed or secreted into the circulation in both normal and disease states. However, the ability to exploit this knowledge for use in clinical medicine has only recently been made possible through the advent of new technologies. Currently, cell-free DNA is being developed as a "real-time liquid biopsy" biomarker to help guide clinical decisions in diverse fields such as prenatal screening, cancer, and solid organ transplantation. The ability of cell-free circulating tumor DNA to be measured quantitatively and qualitatively presents great opportunities in clinical oncology for using blood to monitor tumor burden and assess response to therapies. Here we provide a short review of historic and recent studies demonstrating the clinical potential of detecting and measuring cell-free DNA, with a specific focus on the use of circulating tumor DNA in oncology and cancer management.

Keywords Cancer • Circulating tumor DNA • Plasma tumor DNA • ptDNA • Liquid biopsy

Introduction

Cell-free DNA (cfDNA) is fragmented DNA shed by apoptotic or necrotic cells, as well as actively secreted by both normal and cancerous cells, which can be isolated from secretions, excretions, and bodily fluids [1–3]. The existence of cfDNA was first reported by Mandel and Metais in 1948 [4], but not associated with disease

K. Kyker-Snowman
The Sidney Kimmel Comprehensive Cancer Center, The Johns Hopkins University School of Medicine, 1650 Orleans Street, CRBI Room 116, Baltimore, MD 21287, USA
e-mail: kkykers1@jhmi.edu

B.H. Park (✉)
The Sidney Kimmel Comprehensive Cancer Center, The Johns Hopkins University School of Medicine, 1650 Orleans Street, CRBI Room 151, Baltimore, MD 21287, USA

Department of Chemical and Biomolecular Engineering, The Johns Hopkins University, 1650 Orleans Street, CRBI Room 151, Baltimore, MD 21287, USA
e-mail: bpark2@jhmi.edu

© Springer International Publishing AG 2017
M. Cristofanilli (ed.), *Liquid Biopsies in Solid Tumors*, Cancer Drug Discovery and Development, DOI 10.1007/978-3-319-50956-3_6

until Leon et al. reported a correlation with cancer in 1977 [5]. Early studies attempted to use total levels of cfDNA as a general cancer marker but met with limited success due to lack of sensitivity and specificity. As sample collection methods and technologies for analysis have improved, clinical applications of this biological resource have become a rapidly evolving area of research.

As a minimally invasive biomarker for health and disease, cfDNA has been explored in many fields including but not limited to oncology [2, 6–12], fetal medicine [13–15], organ transplantation rejection monitoring [16], Parkinson's disease detection [17], and assessment of toxicity during chemotherapy [18]. Methods to analyze cfDNA have been equally diverse, including quantitative PCR [19], exome sequencing [9], and epigenetic analyses [20] to name a few. Each technology for measuring cfDNA has advantages and limitations, often dictated by the particular need or application. Overall, cfDNA has the potential to positively impact patient outcomes in clinical medicine as a mechanism of minimally invasive monitoring, allowing for early detection of disease, assessment of response to therapies, and timely intervention with available treatments.

For clinical oncology, the ability to detect tumor-specific cfDNA has many potential high-impact applications. This is especially true when discussing possible uses of cfDNA for treating solid tumors, where liquid biopsies could prove invaluable for assessing disease similar to the use of blood for diagnosing, characterizing, and guiding treatment decisions for hematologic malignancies such as leukemias. The ability to use cfDNA as a liquid biopsy for cancer relies upon one fundamental premise that all cancers are a disease of altered DNA. This has afforded the advent of targeted therapies to attack tumor-specific mutant proteins, but can also be exploited now for diagnostic purposes. Thus, it is currently recognized that the accumulation of somatic alterations in an evolving tumor cell population includes mutations, translocations, amplifications, gene loss, and epigenetic changes. Collectively, these DNA modifications and alterations give each tumor a select set of tumor-specific variations against a background of normal DNA from other tissues. Because all cells, normal and tumor, shed DNA into the circulation, in general there is a relatively low abundance of tumor-specific cfDNA in the total cfDNA population, with the exception of select cases in metastatic disease. Thus, detection of tumor-specific cfDNA requires highly sensitive techniques, able to discriminate a small minority population of DNA, for example a single base-pair change, compared to the majority of wild-type DNA sequences. In general, one can view tumor-specific cfDNA as biomarkers, with the capacity to be used for early detection and prevention, assessing minimal residual disease to guide additional (adjuvant) therapies for early-stage disease, and monitoring tumor burden and response to therapies for early- and late-stage disease. Importantly, the concept of liquid biopsies allows for a relatively noninvasive method of repeat serial sampling for frequent disease assessment. Moreover, the ability to identify specific drug-sensitizing or resistance mutations in the blood of cancer patients also presents the opportunity to replace standard tissue biopsies, which can often be difficult or impossible to obtain, for assessing a predictive marker for therapeutic response. Although a number of studies have supported these concepts, the use of cfDNA for clinical management is still in its infancy, and requires rigorous prospective validation studies that will demonstrate the use of this promising analyte to guide clinical decision making.

Sources of cfDNA

Due to various nomenclature used throughout the literature, here we first define specific terminology. As described above, cfDNA describes the cell-free DNA that exists in the circulation or other bodily compartments, and is comprised of DNA that is shed or excreted generally as small fragmented pieces of genomic DNA. Circulating DNA, on the other hand, specifically refers to cfDNA that is within bodily fluids, including saliva, lymph, blood (plasma or serum), urine, and other liquid components of the body (Fig. 6.1). This circulating DNA is largely derived from normal cells, but in the case of cancer patients there are cancer DNA molecules present in circulating DNA, due to shedding of this material from cancerous cells, and this is often referred to as circulating tumor DNA or ctDNA. However, it is now evident that not all ctDNA is equivalent in terms of how much tumor DNA is present, with variation between serum, plasma, as well as cerebral spinal fluid (CSF) depending on the location and type of tumor [21, 22]. Thus, because plasma

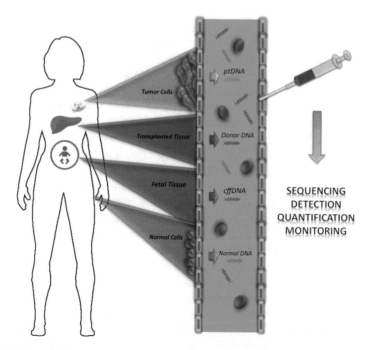

Fig. 6.1 Schematic of varying types of cell-free DNA secreted into the circulation. *ptDNA* plasma tumor DNA, *cffDNA* cell-free fetal DNA

is generally thought to be a superior analyte over serum [23], we refer to circulating plasma tumor DNA as ptDNA for specificity and clarity. The actual amount of cfDNA in individuals is highly variable, but generally is in the range of nanograms per milliliter of blood.

When considering the use of blood for ptDNA analysis, important factors need to be taken into account. These factors include degradation of ptDNA over time, and contamination of ptDNA by genomic DNA due to cell lysis after venipuncture, causing further dilution of an already low-abundant ptDNA fraction, and potentially decreasing sensitivity of any given assay. Cellular lysis is particularly problematic when using serum for ctDNA analysis, since serum is derived from clotted blood, which will generally result in significant cell lysis. Contamination due to cellular DNA can be prevented by rapid processing of blood, using double-centrifugation protocols to separate plasma within 1–2 h after blood acquisition. However, in cases where this is impractical or not feasible, various cell-stabilizing reagents have been effective in preventing cell lysis and preserving the integrity of ptDNA [24].

Technologies to Measure ctDNA/ptDNA

The ability to measure ptDNA holds great promise for diagnosing and monitoring cancer, and in particular the ability to perform serial blood sampling would afford an easy and rapid method of tracking disease. Indeed it was initially appreciated that total levels of cfDNA are often increased with progression of metastatic cancer [3], suggesting simple quantification as a potential biomarker. However, the measurable increase in cfDNA levels that occurs with trauma, inflammation, and other chronic illnesses mandated improvements in the specificity of detection methods for ctDNA. Over the past decade, various technologies have evolved for ctDNA identification and measurement. For example, real-time PCR has been used to measure total levels of cfDNA, and can provide relative quantification of the amount of ctDNA using probes specific for mutations or other alterations [2]. However, the limited sensitivity of real-time PCR for quantification of ctDNA presents challenges, particularly in cancer patients' blood, where mutations are generally present at low allelic frequencies. Thus, rare mutation detection technologies have emerged and continue to evolve. Among newer technologies, digital PCR and next-generation sequencing (NGS) are among the most common techniques employed. Even within these two broad categories, different platforms and methods have been developed with varying sensitivities and specificities. These include the two digital PCR methods beads, emulsions, amplifications, magnetics (BEAMing) and droplet digital PCR (ddPCR), as well as various amplicon-based NGS methods with specialized bioinformatics analysis including tagged amplicon sequencing [25], SAFESeqs [26], and duplex sequencing [27]. Although comparatively expensive, the advantage of NGS is the assessment of multiple genes in the same sample without a priori knowledge of the mutations present. In contrast, digital PCR, including ddPCR, utilizes regionally specific primers and probes to query for a specific mutation of interest and microfluidic partitioning to give a highly sensitive output of binary detection that can then be quantified [10, 19]. Although ddPCR has the disadvantage of querying only for specific mutations, i.e., mutation detection rather than discovery, the key advantages of ddPCR are its relative inexpensive cost per assay, rapid turnaround time, and no requirement for bioinformatics analysis. Some examples of studies using various technologies are described below.

Concordance Studies

In order for liquid biopsies to be validated, there must first be a demonstration that the mutations in blood reflect mutations in the patient's tumor. This notion has proven more complex than originally thought, since there is now widespread recognition of tumor heterogeneity, that is, high degrees of clonal heterogeneity within a primary tumor and metastatic sites of disease [28]. Thus, it is unclear what should be considered the gold standard for mutation detection: a single-site biopsy that is prone to sample selection versus blood that in theory acts as a reservoir for all cancer cells, yet requires ultrasensitive technologies owing to the fact that most cfDNA is derived from normal cells. Despite these nuances, earlier and more recent studies confirm the notion that in general, concordance between tumor tissue mutations and ctDNA is high. Variability arises due to type of cancer examined, as well as differences in and preparation of analytes used (serum versus plasma and processing of plasma), as well as the time between tissue and blood acquisition [29].

One of the first concordance studies performed between cancer tissues and ctDNA used amplification refractory mutation system (ARMS), a method utilizing allele-specific PCR and fluorescent oligonucleotide Scorpion probes for mutation detection, measuring plasma-, serum-, and tumor tissue-derived DNA [8, 30]. In this study Board et al. showed a high concordance (95%) with ARMS measuring *PIK3CA* mutations, comparing plasma-derived ctDNA with corresponding breast tumor tissue samples. This concordance rate also takes into account the concordance between wild-type *PIK3CA* tumors and corresponding blood samples. However, the sensitivity for finding a *PIK3CA* mutation in ctDNA if the tumor was mutation positive, described as a "pickup" rate, was 80% [8]. Intriguingly, this group demonstrated that in a head-to-head comparison, serum samples had lower concordance and sensitivity than corresponding plasma samples from the same patients. This lower sensitivity could possibly be attributable to blood cell lysis with resultant genomic DNA contamination and/or the lower limit of sensitivity for this assay. In addition, mutations in ctDNA were only found in advanced metastatic patients, and no mutations were detectable in early-stage breast cancer patients. Although promising, ARMS is somewhat limited by the cost of Scorpion probes and their design requirements and no true quantification, and has not seen widespread adoption since the advent of digital PCR and NGS technologies.

Another major concordance study was also performed in metastatic breast cancer patients, both retrospectively and prospectively using BEAMing, a digital PCR technology as mentioned above. BEAMing utilizes specific, bead-bound primers for selective amplification of mutant versus wild-type DNA by emulsion-based PCR [31]. Mutation- and wild-type-specific fluorescently labeled hybridization probes are then used after breaking open the emulsions for flow cytometry-based identification of mutant populations that are then quantified. BEAMing was employed by Higgins et al. to demonstrate 100% concordance for *PIK3CA* mutations in ptDNA versus genomic DNA isolated from FFPE tumor tissue samples when the two were obtained contemporaneously [32], both retrospectively and prospectively. However, in the prospective cohort, the group showed that concordance was significantly less between tumor and blood samples when they were obtained greater than 3 years apart [32]. The relative concordance in this study demonstrates both the accuracy of BEAMing and the importance of assessing mutation status in the context of current, rather than archived, samples, due to the potential for rapid evolution in the heterogeneous population of tumor cells.

Another concordance study has been performed in metastatic breast cancer patients called tagged amplicon sequencing (TAm-Seq), which is a high-throughput method of multiplexing known common "hotspot" cancer gene loci in an NGS platform using a PCR amplification strategy for enrichment. This allows for the identification and quantification of multiple DNA variants as shown by Dawson et al. using ptDNA from metastatic breast cancer patients [33]. In this study, the group performed serial analysis of ptDNA by personalized assays of TAm-Seq and digital PCR, and showed that monitoring of ptDNA was superior in measuring response to therapies and tumor burden compared to known protein biomarkers and circulating tumor cells (CTCs). Because the half-life of ptDNA is estimated to be ~1–2 h [2], ptDNA lends itself as an ideal marker for measuring response to therapies. This same group then demonstrated concordance between metastatic biopsies and ptDNA using whole-exome NGS, though in a relatively small sample size [34]. Importantly, there were instances of discordant results, with mutations found only in tissues and conversely, exclusively in blood, highlighting limitations of both analytes and perhaps the techniques used for these studies, i.e., whole-exome NGS on blood, which may not be as sensitive due to the relatively lower depth of coverage for any given locus.

Given the importance of targeted therapies for certain mutations found in specific cancers such as non-small-cell lung cancers, liquid biopsies have also been of keen interest to identify not only molecular predictors of drug sensitivity, but also resistance. For example, Wei et al. monitored the erlotinib/gefitinib resistance conferring T790M *EGFR* mutation in 50 metastatic non-small-cell lung cancer patients by digital PCR [35]. They found 82% concordance with tissue biopsies, and importantly described patients without T790M mutations that then developed progressive, resistant disease while on EGFR inhibitors and were subsequently found to have the T790M mutations in both blood and newly biopsied tissues.

A recent study of breast cancer patients compared ptDNA and metastatic tissue samples using NGS with a limited cancer gene panel [36]. Although limited by a small sample size (17 patients), the majority of samples had concordance between tissue and blood samples, though again there were instances of mutations found only in tissues and only in blood. The authors concluded that plasma could be prospectively tested as an alternative to tissue for mutational testing. Finally, other sources of ctDNA have also been subjected to concordance studies. Although primary brain tumors are not felt to "shed" DNA into the bloodstream at the same level of non-CNS tumors, recent studies have demonstrated concordance of mutations in primary brain tumors with cerebral spinal fluid (CSF). Bettegowda and colleagues showed that in patients with primary brain cancers, somatic alterations in tumor could be found in CSF in 74% of cases [22]. A more recent study using NGS demonstrated high concordance of genetic alterations between the cell pellets within the CSF, and the cell-free component of CSF using the IMPACT 341 cancer gene panel NGS assay [37]. Collectively these studies highlight that the concordance between cancer tissues and cells with cfDNA is quite high, and it is likely that ctDNA offers a more easily obtainable analyte for mutation discovery and detection that is reflective of the patient's cancer and in some cases more comprehensive due to tumor heterogeneity within and between sites of metastatic disease.

Clinical Applications: Prevention and Screening

Earlier detection and diagnosis of cancer using ctDNA is a highly anticipated area of active research, as earlier detection and treatment is generally associated with improved patient outcomes. However, high levels of sensitivity and specificity are required for screening in order to assure acceptable limits of false-negative and false-positive results. Additionally, screening tests for cancer should generally be proven to reduce the morbidity and/or mortality of the cancer being screened for. It should be noted that very few screening modalities for early cancer detection and diagnosis have met these benchmarks. Conversely, earlier detection of cancer raises the conundrum in clinical medicine of "overdiagnosis," resulting in further testing with associated costs and anxiety, and increased use of scans and biopsy, and ultimately producing the need for long-term studies that definitively prove that early detection affects overall mortality, i.e., the intervention saves lives above and beyond not using the screening test. Although historically the lack of sensitivity and specificity for cancer detection limited "useful" screening methods, improved technologies have led to the current unsettled issues of what should be considered standard-of-care practice for screening tests such as mammography, prostate-specific antigen (PSA) testing, and colonoscopy. Given the complexities and barriers needed to bring widespread adoption for any cancer-screening test, only a limited number of studies have begun to address the use of ctDNA for early detection and prevention, including a small study using cervical fluid ctDNA for endometrial and ovarian cancer detection [38], and a small study linking the integrity of plasma DNA to the progression of early-stage prostate cancer [39]. Nonetheless, the use of ctDNA may be helpful as an adjunct test to primary screening tools in certain high-risk populations. For example, one could envision that serial blood draws to detect new mutations in ptDNA after an abnormal mammogram, PSA, or colonoscopy could be used to increase the detection specificity for indeterminate lesions detected on annual screens.

Clinical Applications: Early-Stage Cancer

Perhaps one of the most challenging unmet needs in clinical oncology is the current paradigm of adjuvant therapies leading to "overtreatment" for early-stage disease. Breast cancer, given its high incidence, is a prime example of this conundrum. Although it is well accepted that additional systemic therapies such as chemotherapy, HER2-directed therapies, and endocrine therapies have significantly improved disease-free survival and overall survival after local therapies such as surgery and radiation, it is also well accepted that the majority of early-stage breast cancer patients who receive these do not need or benefit from these therapies since they are already cured. Because there is no reliable method of detecting patients with microscopic minimal residual disease after surgery, i.e., the patients at highest risk for relapse, patients with early-stage disease in routine clinical practice go on to receive additional adjuvant systemic therapies after local therapies. While this paradigm clearly cures additional patients and overall leads to more positive than negative outcomes, it is acknowledged that such an approach leads to a small but significant percentage of patients who suffer from short- and long-term consequences of adjuvant therapies, including death. Thus, a technology that could measure microscopic residual disease may afford the opportunity to make informed clinical decisions regarding the need for adjuvant therapies for each individual patient.

Thus far, the majority of ptDNA studies have been performed retrospectively and in metastatic patients. To address the conundrum of overtreatment in early-stage breast cancer, Beaver et al. performed a prospective study comparing Sanger sequencing of FFPE primary breast tumor samples to mutation detection by ddPCR in the same primary breast tumor tissue as well as contemporaneously obtained ptDNA samples in early-stage patients before surgery [6]. This was one of the first studies to utilize ddPCR, which is an automated high-throughput method of digital PCR akin to BEAMing, though the emulsions are uniformly synthesized using automated microfluidics, and detection by fluorescent-based probes occurs within the "droplets" foregoing the need to break open emulsions for mutation analysis. In this study, Beaver et al. queried only for the two most common *PIK3CA* mutations, E545K and H1047R, in 30 breast tumors, demonstrating concordant mutation detection before surgery with a sensitivity of 93.3% and a specificity of 100%. Mutation detection of ptDNA after surgery was also carried out, and in the absence of clinically evident disease, ptDNA was also detected for five patients, with one patient progressing rapidly after completing all standard-of-care treatments. Further study is needed to determine the prognostic power of postsurgical ptDNA detection by ddPCR, but clearly this proof of principle establishes the feasibility of detecting minimal residual disease that can result in recurrent incurable metastatic disease. A recent study by Garcia-Murillas et al. examining early-stage breast cancer patients undergoing neoadjuvant therapy yielded similar results, with ddPCR used to detect ptDNA prior to overt clinical recurrence [40]. Additionally, a retrospective analysis of early-stage breast cancer patients who relapsed also suggests that persistent ptDNA after standard-of-care therapies is a prognostic marker for relapse [41].

Clinical Applications: Metastatic Cancer

The ability to assay for cancer mutations in ptDNA in metastatic cancer patients also holds promise for great clinical utility. For example, lung cancer patients who may not have easily accessible lesions could potentially use ptDNA to assess mutations in *EGFR* that predict for sensitivity to EGFR kinase inhibitors [42–44], as well as *EGFR* mutations that predict for resistance to these same therapies [45, 46]. Similarly, ptDNA could be used to serially monitor metastatic colorectal cancer patients for the emergence of *KRAS* mutations that predict for resistance to EGFR antibody-based therapies [47, 48]. In addition, although copy number assessments can be challenging in ptDNA, there are studies that suggest that this is feasible. For example, *HER2* amplification for breast and possibly other cancers may one day be assayed through the use of blood [49], providing an opportunity for clinical utility in metastatic breast cancers, as well as select gastrointestinal malignancies.

A potential useful concept for ptDNA is the idea of using the quantity of ptDNA in a patient's blood as a measure of overall tumor growth and response to therapy. One could envision using a small panel of cancer genes to quantitatively assess the levels of mutations in a metastatic patient's blood and then after one dose of therapy determine if there is a response. Current practice for most solid metastatic malignancies is to wait for 2–3 cycles (often 3–4 months) before reassessing response using imaging. Although standard of care, this often results in progressive disease and useless therapies for a significant amount of time. Therefore the potential utility of liquid biopsies in this setting would be to change therapies earlier based upon ptDNA response after a single dose of therapy. This approach could also be financially incentivized, since there would be no need to pay for additional cycles of ineffective therapies. To this end, Tie et al. recently completed a small proof-of-principle study in metastatic colorectal cancer patients that suggest that such a strategy is feasible [50]. More research in this promising arena is currently under way.

ptDNA may also serve as a useful marker of prognosis for metastatic patients, since the amount of ptDNA is a reflection of tumor burden. For example, Wyatt et al. serially profiled ptDNA in men with castration-resistant metastatic prostate cancer to assess for copy number and mutations in androgen receptor (AR) along with targeted sequencing of 19 genes through subsequent therapies [51]. They found that the presence and/or emergence of AR alterations and *RB1* loss was associated with a worse prognosis in this group of patients, suggesting that ptDNA could be used to identify markers of prognosis and perhaps resistance to certain therapies. Similarly, Dawson et al. demonstrated that ptDNA has prognostic value in metastatic breast cancer patients, with a wider dynamic range than CTCs [33]. Although perhaps expected given that ptDNA directly correlates with tumor burden, these and other studies convincingly demonstrate that ptDNA can be used as prognostic bio-markers in metastatic disease.

Finally, an emerging concept that readily lends itself as a ptDNA diagnostic test is the recent discovery of *ESR1* mutations in metastatic breast cancer. Several groups have reported that mutations in the ligand-binding domain within the estrogen receptor-alpha gene, *ESR1*, can confer constitutive receptor activation and resistance to endocrine therapies [52–56]. Due to the small number of patients evaluated in most of these studies, along with the problem of tumor heterogeneity and thus single-site biopsy, ptDNA analysis for *ESR1* mutations might reveal insights into the true frequency of these mutations in metastatic breast cancer patients who progress on endocrine therapies. One of the first studies to use both retrospective and prospective cohorts to address this was recently published by Chu et al. [10]. In this study, the authors analyzed ptDNA via ddPCR to detect *ESR1* mutations in plasma samples from metastatic breast cancer patients that had progressed on endocrine therapies [10]. Although this study cannot be considered conclusive due to the small sample size, the authors did show that ddPCR could detect *ESR1* mutations in ptDNA, and could detect additional mutations not identified by NGS of corresponding metastatic tumor tissues. Similarly, Sefrioui et al. retrospectively tested plasma and corresponding tumor samples from a small number of patients with metastatic breast cancer and prior exposure to aromatase inhibitors [57]. A higher frequency of *ESR1* mutations compared to sequencing of tissue was also detected in this study, and in two patients, serial monitoring predicted for disease recurrence. In a similar vein, Guttery et al. used targeted NGS and ddPCR to demonstrate the emergence of *ESR1* mutant clones, suggesting that monitoring of ctDNA could be an early marker of resistance [58]. Moreover, Shiovan et al. showed that *ESR1* mutations appeared at a higher frequency in patients progressing on aromatase inhibitors in metastatic patients compared to patients receiving therapy for early-stage disease in the adjuvant setting [59]. Finally, two recent studies suggest that certain endocrine therapies such as fulvestrant with or without the new CDK4/6 inhibitor, palbociclib, may be able to overcome *ESR1* resistance mutations [60, 61]. Collectively these studies support the idea that the use of ptDNA can identify *ESR1* mutations with improved sensitivity over tissue biopsies due to tumor heterogeneity, and that these mutations are markers of endocrine therapy resistance. Due to the ever-increasing therapeutic options for patients with metastatic estrogen receptor-positive disease, these results suggest that ptDNA detection of *ESR1* mutations could inform future therapeutic decision that would then lead to improved clinical outcomes.

Conclusions

Circulating ptDNA has enormous potential as a liquid biopsy to improve early diagnosis, aid in adjuvant therapy decisions, and guide decisions in metastatic disease in terms of therapeutic predictive efficacy and prognosis. Early studies have demonstrated a consistent and fairly high concordance of ptDNA with tumor biopsy sequencing, and the ability to detect mutations that can predict for sensitivity or resistance to targeted therapies. Improvements in the technologies used to identify and measure ptDNA indicate that ptDNA monitoring may have utility in mutation detection and assessing progressive metastatic cancer and response to therapies in real time. Further studies including prospective validation of ptDNA are needed in order to translate this nascent field from exciting laboratory research to actual clinical tests with proven utility. Ultimately, liquid biopsies incorporating ptDNA analysis could completely change the way oncologists make informed decisions, allowing them to select the most effective therapies for their patients.

Acknowledgments This work was supported by the Avon Foundation and the Canney Foundation. We would also like to thank and acknowledge the support of NIH P30 CA006973, the Eddie and Sandy Garcia Charitable Foundation, the Commonwealth Foundation, the Santa Fe Foundation, the Marcie and Ellen Foundation, the Helen Golde Trust, and the Robin Page/Lebor Foundation. None of the funding sources influenced the design, interpretation, or submission of this manuscript.

Disclosures B.H.P. is a member of the scientific advisory boards for Horizon Discovery, LTD and Loxo Oncology; is a consultant for Foundation Medicine, Inc.; and has research contracts with Genomic Health, Inc. and Foundation Medicine, Inc. Under separate licensing agreements between Horizon Discovery, LTD and the Johns Hopkins University, B.H.P. is entitled to a share of royalties received by the university on sales of products. The terms of this arrangement are being managed by the Johns Hopkins University, in accordance with its conflict of interest policies. B.H.P. also has ownership interest in Loxo Oncology. K.K.-S. declares no potential conflicts.

References

1. Kohler C, Barekati Z, Radpour R et al (2011) Cell-free DNA in the circulation as a potential cancer biomarker. Anticancer Res 31:2623–2628
2. Diehl F, Schmidt K, Choti MA et al (2008) Circulating mutant DNA to assess tumor dynamics. Nat Med 14:985–990
3. Heitzer E, Ulz P, Geigl JB (2015) Circulating tumor DNA as a liquid biopsy for cancer. Clin Chem 61:112–123
4. Mandel P, Metais P (1948) C R Seances Soc Biol Fil 142:241–243
5. Leon SA, Shapiro B, Sklaroff DM et al (1977) Free DNA in the serum of cancer patients and the effect of therapy. Cancer Res 37:646–650
6. Beaver JA, Jelovac D, Balukrishna S et al (2014) Detection of cancer DNA in plasma of patients with early-stage breast cancer. Clin Cancer Res 20:2643–2650
7. Benesova L, Belsanova B, Suchanek S et al (2013) Mutation-based detection and monitoring of cell-free tumor DNA in peripheral blood of cancer patients. Anal Biochem 433:227–234
8. Board RE, Wardley AM, Dixon JM et al (2010) Detection of PIK3CA mutations in circulating free DNA in patients with breast cancer. Breast Cancer Res Treat 120:461–467
9. Butler TM, Johnson-Camacho K, Peto M et al (2015) Exome sequencing of cell-free DNA from metastatic cancer patients identifies clinically actionable mutations distinct from primary disease. PLoS One 10:e0136407
10. Chu D, Paoletti C, Gersch C et al (2015) ESR1 mutations in circulating plasma tumor DNA from metastatic breast cancer patients. Clin Cancer Res 22(4):993

11. Chen WW, Balaj L, Liau LM et al (2013) BEAMing and droplet digital PCR analysis of mutant IDH1 mRNA in glioma patient serum and cerebrospinal fluid extracellular vesicles. Mol Ther Nucleic Acids 2:e109
12. Kin C, Kidess E, Poultsides GA et al (2013) Colorectal cancer diagnostics: biomarkers, cell-free DNA, circulating tumor cells and defining heterogeneous populations by single-cell analysis. Expert Rev Mol Diagn 13:581–599
13. Karakas B, Qubbaj W, Al-Hassan S et al (2015) Noninvasive digital detection of fetal DNA in plasma of 4-week-pregnant women following in vitro fertilization and embryo transfer. PLoS One 10:e0126501
14. Park HJ, Shim SS, Cha DH (2015) Combined screening for early detection of pre-eclampsia. Int J Mol Sci 16:17952–17974
15. Stokowski R, Wang E, White K et al (2015) Clinical performance of non-invasive prenatal testing (NIPT) using targeted cell-free DNA analysis in maternal plasma with microarrays or next generation sequencing (NGS) is consistent across multiple controlled clinical studies. Prenat Diagn 35(12):1243
16. Gielis EM, Ledeganck KJ, De Winter BY et al (2015) Cell-free DNA: an upcoming biomarker in transplantation. Am J Transplant 15:2541–2551
17. Pyle A, Brennan R, Kurzawa-Akanbi M et al (2015) Reduced CSF mitochondrial DNA is a biomarker for early-stage Parkinson's disease. Ann Neurol 78(6):1000
18. Christenson ES, James T, Agrawal V et al (2015) Use of biomarkers for the assessment of chemotherapy-induced cardiac toxicity. Clin Biochem 48:223–235
19. Hindson CM, Chevillet JR, Briggs HA et al (2013) Absolute quantification by droplet digital PCR versus analog real-time PCR. Nat Methods 10:1003–1005
20. Legendre C, Gooden GC, Johnson K et al (2015) Whole-genome bisulfite sequencing of cell-free DNA identifies signature associated with metastatic breast cancer. Clin Epigenetics 7:100
21. Beaver JA, Park BH (2015) Detecting plasma tumor DNA in early-stage breast cancer—reply. Clin Cancer Res 21:3570
22. Wang Y, Springer S, Zhang M et al (2015) Detection of tumor-derived DNA in cerebrospinal fluid of patients with primary tumors of the brain and spinal cord. Proc Natl Acad Sci U S A 112:9704–9709
23. El Messaoudi S, Rolet F, Mouliere F et al (2013) Circulating cell free DNA: preanalytical considerations. Clin Chim Acta 424:222–230
24. Toro PV, Erlanger B, Beaver JA et al (2015) Comparison of cell stabilizing blood collection tubes for circulating plasma tumor DNA. Clin Biochem 48(15):993
25. Forshew T, Murtaza M, Parkinson C et al (2012) Noninvasive identification and monitoring of cancer mutations by targeted deep sequencing of plasma DNA. Sci Transl Med 4:136ra68
26. Kinde I, Wu J, Papadopoulos N et al (2011) Detection and quantification of rare mutations with massively parallel sequencing. Proc Natl Acad Sci U S A 108:9530–9535
27. Schmitt MW, Kennedy SR, Salk JJ et al (2012) Detection of ultra-rare mutations by next-generation sequencing. Proc Natl Acad Sci U S A 109:14508–14513
28. Gerlinger M, Rowan AJ, Horswell S et al (2012) Intratumor heterogeneity and branched evolution revealed by multiregion sequencing. N Engl J Med 366:883–892
29. Bettegowda C, Sausen M, Leary RJ et al (2014) Detection of circulating tumor DNA in early- and late-stage human malignancies. Sci Transl Med 6:224ra224
30. Board RE, Thelwell NJ, Ravetto PF et al (2008) Multiplexed assays for detection of mutations in PIK3CA. Clin Chem 54:757–760
31. Dressman D, Yan H, Traverso G et al (2003) Transforming single DNA molecules into fluorescent magnetic particles for detection and enumeration of genetic variations. Proc Natl Acad Sci U S A 100:8817–8822
32. Higgins MJ, Jelovac D, Barnathan E et al (2012) Detection of tumor PIK3CA status in metastatic breast cancer using peripheral blood. Clin Cancer Res 18:3462–3469
33. Dawson SJ, Tsui DW, Murtaza M et al (2013) Analysis of circulating tumor DNA to monitor metastatic breast cancer. N Engl J Med 368:1199–1209
34. Murtaza M, Dawson SJ, Tsui DW et al (2013) Non-invasive analysis of acquired resistance to cancer therapy by sequencing of plasma DNA. Nature 497:108–112

35. Wei Z, Shah N, Deng C et al (2016) Circulating DNA addresses cancer monitoring in non small cell lung cancer patients for detection and capturing the dynamic changes of the disease. Springerplus 5:531
36. Rothé F, Laes J-F, Lambrechts D, Smeets D, Vincent D, Maetens M, Fumagalli D, Michiels S, Stylianos D, Moerman C, Detiffe J-P, Larsimont D, Awada A, Piccart M, Sotiriou C, Ignatiadis M (2014) Plasma circulating tumor DNA as an alternative to metastatic biopsies for mutational analysis in breast cancer. Ann Oncol 25(10):1959
37. Pentsova EI, Shah RH, Tang J et al (2016) Evaluating cancer of the central nervous system through next-generation sequencing of cerebrospinal fluid. J Clin Oncol 34(20):2404
38. Kinde I, Bettegowda C, Wang Y et al (2013) Evaluation of DNA from the Papanicolaou test to detect ovarian and endometrial cancers. Sci Transl Med 5:167ra164
39. Delgado PO, Alves BC, Gehrke Fde S et al (2013) Characterization of cell-free circulating DNA in plasma in patients with prostate cancer. Tumour Biol 34:983–986
40. Garcia-Murillas I, Schiavon G, Weigelt B et al (2015) Mutation tracking in circulating tumor DNA predicts relapse in early breast cancer. Sci Transl Med 7:302ra133
41. Olsson E, Winter C, George A et al (2015) Serial monitoring of circulating tumor DNA in patients with primary breast cancer for detection of occult metastatic disease. EMBO Mol Med 7:1034–1047
42. Lynch TJ, Bell DW, Sordella R et al (2004) Activating mutations in the epidermal growth factor receptor underlying responsiveness of non-small-cell lung cancer to gefitinib. N Engl J Med 350:2129–2139
43. Paez JG, Janne PA, Lee JC et al (2004) EGFR mutations in lung cancer: correlation with clinical response to gefitinib therapy. Science 304:1497–1500
44. Pao W, Miller V, Zakowski M et al (2004) EGF receptor gene mutations are common in lung cancers from "never smokers" and are associated with sensitivity of tumors to gefitinib and erlotinib. Proc Natl Acad Sci U S A 101:13306–13311
45. Taniguchi K, Uchida J, Nishino K et al (2011) Quantitative detection of EGFR mutations in circulating tumor DNA derived from lung adenocarcinomas. Clin Cancer Res 17:7808–7815
46. Pao W, Miller VA, Politi KA et al (2005) Acquired resistance of lung adenocarcinomas to gefitinib or erlotinib is associated with a second mutation in the EGFR kinase domain. PLoS Med 2:e73
47. Siravegna G, Mussolin B, Buscarino M et al (2015) Clonal evolution and resistance to EGFR blockade in the blood of colorectal cancer patients. Nat Med 21:795–801
48. Misale S, Yaeger R, Hobor S et al (2012) Emergence of KRAS mutations and acquired resistance to anti-EGFR therapy in colorectal cancer. Nature 486:532–536
49. Gevensleben H, Garcia-Murillas I, Graeser MK et al (2013) Noninvasive detection of HER2 amplification with plasma DNA digital PCR. Clin Cancer Res 19:3276–3284
50. Tie J, Kinde I, Wang Y et al (2015) Circulating tumor DNA as an early marker of therapeutic response in patients with metastatic colorectal cancer. Ann Oncol 26(8):1715
51. Wyatt AW, Azad AA, Volik SV et al (2016) Genomic alterations in cell-free DNA and enzalutamide resistance in castration-resistant prostate cancer. JAMA Oncol 2(12):1598
52. Li S, Shen D, Shao J et al (2013) Endocrine-therapy-resistant ESR1 variants revealed by genomic characterization of breast-cancer-derived xenografts. Cell Rep 4:1116–1130
53. Merenbakh-Lamin K, Ben-Baruch N, Yeheskel A et al (2013) D538G mutation in estrogen receptor-alpha: A novel mechanism for acquired endocrine resistance in breast cancer. Cancer Res 73:6856–6864
54. Robinson DR, Wu YM, Vats P et al (2013) Activating ESR1 mutations in hormone-resistant metastatic breast cancer. Nat Genet 45:1446–1451
55. Toy W, Shen Y, Won H et al (2013) ESR1 ligand-binding domain mutations in hormone-resistant breast cancer. Nat Genet 45:1439–1445
56. Jeselsohn R, Yelensky R, Buchwalter G et al (2014) Emergence of constitutively active estrogen receptor-alpha mutations in pretreated advanced estrogen receptor-positive breast cancer. Clin Cancer Res 20:1757–1767

57. Sefrioui D, Perdrix A, Sarafan-Vasseur N et al (2015) Short report: monitoring ESR1 muta-
    tions by circulating tumor DNA in aromatase inhibitor resistant metastatic breast cancer. Int
    J Cancer 137:2513–2519
58. Guttery DS, Page K, Hills A et al (2015) Noninvasive detection of activating estrogen receptor
    1 (ESR1) mutations in estrogen receptor-positive metastatic breast cancer. Clin Chem
    61:974–982
59. Schiavon G, Hrebien S, Garcia-Murillas I et al (2015) Analysis of ESR1 mutation in circulating
    tumor DNA demonstrates evolution during therapy for metastatic breast cancer. Sci Transl
    Med 7:313ra182
60. Spoerke JM, Gendreau S, Walter K et al (2016) Heterogeneity and clinical significance of
    ESR1 mutations in ER-positive metastatic breast cancer patients receiving fulvestrant. Nat
    Commun 7:11579
61. Fribbens C, O'Leary B, Kilburn L et al (2016) Plasma ESR1 mutations and the treatment of
    estrogen receptor-positive advanced breast cancer. J Clin Oncol 34(25):2961

Chapter 7
CTCs and ctDNA: Two Tales of a Complex Biology

Paul W. Dempsey

Abstract A significant interest in the emerging liquid biopsy technologies has been driven by new tools for analysis of nucleic acids and alterations that are associated with cancer. As is so often the case, the gains from new technology come not from the technology itself but from the improved understanding of the biology. Using these tools, data on the detection of tumor-derived cells and tumor-derived fragmented DNA in a blood sample has focused much energy on developing sustainable validated protocols to analyze these samples. The emerging data on cell-free and cell-derived molecular templates supports a complementary analysis of these compartments depending on the sensitivity requirements, nature of the genetic alteration, biomarker needs, and clinical evidence required.

Keywords Liquid biopsy • Circulating biomarkers • Complementary biomarkers • CTC • CtDNA

Introduction

Cancer is a genetic disease [1]. In the simplest model, changes in growth regulation and control, ultimately caused by changes in DNA sequence, generate clones of cells that grow in an unregulated manner [2]. Changes in growth control have allowed for development of therapies that specifically target pathways that become constitutively active, simple examples being inhibition of tyrosine kinase pathways such as Her2 [3] or BCR-ABL [4]. As for most treatment cycles in cancer and the resulting selection process, additional changes and clonal variation ultimately result in tumor clones that escape treatment and metastasize to remote sites possibly quite early in the disease process [5, 6]. It is the metastasis that cause cancer-associated mortality. Therefore, in order to more effectively detect, monitor, and treat cancer, additional tools to monitor disease are being developed. Many of these have focused on the tumor-derived template that can be recovered from blood. Because of the genetic nature of the disease, the molecular fingerprint of cancer is manifest in the

P.W. Dempsey (✉)
Cynvenio Biosystems Inc., Westlake Village, CA, USA
e-mail: pdempsey@cynvenio.com

© Springer International Publishing AG 2017   119
M. Cristofanilli (ed.), *Liquid Biopsies in Solid Tumors*, Cancer Drug Discovery and Development, DOI 10.1007/978-3-319-50956-3_7

DNA recovered either in the circulating cell-free DNA (ccfDNA) compartment or in circulating tumor-derived cells (circulating tumor cells or CTCs). Both of these templates were originally described many decades ago. However both required the development of relatively recent technologies to support their analysis.

Broadly speaking, CTCs and the nucleic acids they contain reflect the mobile, metastatic cell population that is driving the disease [7, 8]. In contrast, ccfDNA is generated by processes associated with apoptosis and necrosis and represents an aggregate of those aspects of the disease that are undergoing these processes [9]. ccfDNA has been the simpler sample to acquire and as such has garnered the greater attention of late due to the lack of molecular options in the CTC compartment. However emerging technologies are changing this. Furthermore, due to the cost-effective broad access to next-generation sequencing (NGS) technologies [10], we can now measure informative DNA molecules and cells by detecting the presence of specific changes associated with cancer. Any process of discovery is limited by the tools we have to examine it. So too is our understanding of tumor-derived template dependent on the technologies we can bring to bear. Therefore, we should examine the technology to understand the biology.

Advantages and Challenges of Blood-Derived Biopsy

The gold standard for molecular analysis of tumor tissue has been biopsy [11–13]. Biopsy sample is generated by surgery or other targeted mechanisms such as core needle sampling. It harvests a population of tumor cells from a single site. The tumor cells having expanded at the one site are related and are the best representation of the related clones that have been selected to grow and expand at that site [14, 15]. While this has produced a great deal of information about basic tumor development, it does not necessarily provide any information about mechanisms of metastasis; just at best the consequences. In contrast, blood tissue monitors all sites in the body. With this mechanism, tumor material from different sites can become distributed in blood. So tumor cells or ccfDNA can be recovered that reflect the entire disease [16]. As such it is a fundamentally different sample mechanism than the gold standard. This is because each cell or DNA fragment is distributed one molecule or one cell at a time and will reflect the disease and its heterogeneity differently. So fundamentally, the analysis of blood-derived template is different from a biopsy-derived sample. Recent data elucidate these differences.

Circulating Tumor Cells

The evidence that populations of cells derived from solid tumors are found in blood stretches all the way back to 1869 when cells with a very similar phenotype to the original cancer were observed in the blood on necropsy [17]. This isolated observation made sense in light of the clinical observations around metastatic cancers; it is the movement of tumor cells to distal sites such as the lung, liver, bone, or brain that are responsible for the associated mortality [18]. Understanding how tumor cells migrate raises many questions. What governs their motility? What is the process of locating to a metastatic site? Are there different cell populations with different mobilities? These are all questions that will shed light on understanding the process by which cancer becomes a lethal disease. To address any of these questions, it is necessary to build a process that allows interrogation of these rare populations of cells.

Early attempts to identify cells of tumor origin were limited to simple observational technologies that relied on pathologic description in cytospin preparations or fluorescence-activated cytometers [19–21]. With occasional rare examples of clear malignancy, these approaches did emphasize one aspect that the field has continued to grapple with: Just what is a tumor cell when it is in blood and how is it to be distinguished from rare or unusual cells that are in blood because of unrelated biological processes? The definition used to identify cells in the blood that are derived from tumor influences the assumptions made about the classes of cells that can be interrogated.

CTCs have all been defined using one of the three experimental approaches. The different approaches have caused some confusion despite the fact that they are in many cases describing overlapping populations of cells. Broadly speaking CTCs have been identified using (1) enumeration, where an immunophenotypic population of cells that is elevated in patients with cancer were characterized and shown to be associated with more aggressive disease [22]; (2) functional, where a population of cells is shown to have the ability to form xenografts in mice or grow ex vivo [23]; and (3) molecular, where a population of cells in blood is shown to bear molecular hallmarks of cancer that can be traced back to one of the tumor sites [24]. These definitions are not mutually exclusive depending on how the experiments are performed. It can be expected that emerging molecular tools will serve to further blur the boundaries between these definitions.

Enumeration: All enumeration technologies leverage the precedent established by the CellSearch platform. This is the only FDA-approved test to count circulating tumor cells. In point of fact, the test actually enumerates epithelial cells using EpCAM to capture cells and antibodies to the intracellular epithelial antigen cytokeratin to detect the cells [25]. DAPI and anti-CD45 reagents are used to confirm the presence of a nucleus and to distinguish white blood cells (WBC). What this definition does not include is any metric that clearly and specifically demonstrates these cells are tumor derived, for instance, by the presence of disease-associated mutations. In the absence of a tumor-specific marker, the utility of these CTCs was established in careful prospective clinical trials. By measuring CTC numbers in patients with metastatic breast cancer and following their outcome, Cristofanilli et al. were able to show that five CTCs recovered from 7.5 mL of blood were prognostic for more rapid progression and worse overall survival [26]. This initial observation has been substantively expanded to much larger studies, all of which have reconfirmed the prognostic value of five CTCs per 7.5 mL [8, 27–29]. In addition, the standardized recovery and detection afforded by CellSearch have been used to demonstrate that as few as one CTC in nonmetastatic breast cancer also has a worse prognosis [30]. CTC number has further been shown to be associated with increased risk and number of metastasis [31]. The same prognostic risk of progression was shown based on enumeration of CTC in both colorectal [32, 33] and prostate cancer [34, 35]. So these data built a platform and reagent-specific definition of a CTC.

Functional: A second approach to defining CTC grew out of an effort to understand which population of cells in a tumor were capable of mediating metastatic events. The rationale was that cells that are capable of establishing metastatic events must have the potential to seed distant sites with very few cells and have the potential to recapitulate all the tumor phenotypes that are found in a metastatic site. The model for the change from localized epithelial to a mobile metastatic cell with a mesenchymal phenotype is referred to as epithelial mesenchymal transition (EMT). Simplistically, EMT reverses the cascade that leads to the development and migration of progenitor stem cells during organ development. As this process is deregulated by the transformation, mobility and dedifferentiation increase. Critically, this process has to work in both directions as when a metastatic cell is mobilized and moves to a new location, a mobility program has to reverse and an epithelial program is needed to establish a new metastatic site [36]. This reversible transitional potential was identified in a population of cells that were EpCAM+, CD44+, and CD24−. These cells were capable of initiating tumor development in immunodeficient NOD mice with as few as 100 cells [37], thus providing a functional definition of a "tumor-initiating cell." This population of tumor-initiating cells has a plastic ability to rapidly alter patterns of expression consistent with a canonical epithelial mesenchymal transition state to a mesenchymal expression pattern as predicted by EMT modeling [38]. Importantly, the convergence of these cells and those characterized by EpCAM enumeration starts to build biological definitions that serve as a Rosetta Stone for a more complete understanding of the relationship between tumor-initiating cells and CTC [39]. This is supported by the transient expression of EMT phenotypes on CTC [40, 41] that are related to prognosis [42].

Molecular: Molecular definitions of tumor cells in blood rely on detection of alterations in the genomic DNA of the cells that can always be associated with the presence of tumor, or are shown to be present in the parent tumor. In the simplest form, this has been shown in cytospins of blood samples where tumor cells can be demonstrated to have hallmarks of cancer as shown by detection of amplified Her2 [43], or AR loci [44] or other evidence of malignancy [45, 46]. Given their rarity, the majority of efforts to demonstrate molecular hallmarks of tumor in CTC come on the back of enrichment platforms. So tumor cells recovered by the CellSearch platform have been shown to include cells with a malignant genotype [47]. Tellingly, in many such analysis the tumor cells are present molecularly as a heterogeneous population whether detected by Her2 amplification or by sequencing for EGFR mutations [48]. This raises two questions: What are these other cells where a malignant genotype was not demonstrated? Are we just not using the correct tools to determine malignancy or are the cells associated with some other aspect of the disease process but contain a normal genome? How are we to understand other enrichment approaches that, by uncoupling from the validated CellSearch definition, are able to enrich different populations of cells?

What Impact Does Technology Have on Our Understanding of CTC

The CellSearch platform is a robust, standardized tool approved to recover rare epithelial cells from a blood sample. However, it does have many challenges. Firstly, the number of events is almost always very low. In fact, while the platform is capable of detecting a single event, the stochastic sampling problem of counting cells at such a low rate is very challenging. The CTC enumeration test for colorectal cancer was approved with only three cells as a prognostic threshold suggesting that in this disease the population of these EpCAM-positive, cytokeratin-expressing cells might be even smaller than in breast and prostate cancer [33]. One result of this is a significant number of samples that have no detectable CTC. For example, in repeated validations of CTC numbers in metastatic breast cancer, typically less than 50% of the samples contain the threshold number of five CTCs [26]. This means that the vast majority of samples contain less than 1 cell/mL. This will always present an engineering challenge in terms of limits of detection.

Largely due to the rarity of this cell population, there emerged a series of competing technologies designed to detect additional numbers of CTCs. These technologies assumed that there were many more cells available in blood than are captured by the CellSearch which is simply less efficient being a batch-based enrichment procedure. In fact, by any measure CellSearch is very efficient at recovery of EpCAM-expressing cells [49, 50]. Therefore, differences in EpCAM capture performance are much more likely to be differences in detection or in defining positive events highlighting the challenge of standardized approaches [51]. When the reagents or the hardware are changed, the classification of recovered cells has to be independently validated if it is different. On this matter, it is noteworthy that cells that meet the definition for CTC using the CellSearch platform can be detected occasionally in normal healthy individuals [26]. Also, in conditions of chronic inflammation, cells that meet the definition of a CTC are regularly detected emphasizing the challenge of cell classification [52]. Therefore, the value of a CellSearch number is closely tied to the prognostic impact that was demonstrated for that platform and emphasizes the care needed to move beyond this definition.

Changing the definition of a CTC comes either from altering the enrichment procedure or the detection definition. For instance, it is possible that the CellSearch platform captures CTCs that express EpCAM but not cytokeratin. These EpCAM-positive cytokeratin-negative events would therefore be missed during the detection step [53]. It was this performance challenge that drove the development of additional technologies to detect the presence of CTC and expand the size of the population. First among these were PCR-based approaches to detect cells in blood that expressed the same detection biomarkers. Cells captured with antibodies against

EpCAM and Muc1 were detected by RT-PCR to detect the presence of EpCAM and Her2 transcripts [54]. While this tool did produce signal in an overlapping population of patients, it was not anymore prognostically sensitive than CellSearch [55]. More to the point, there are populations of cells in healthy normals that have recoverable cells that express transcripts for all of the detection targets including Her2 and EpCAM [56] reinforcing the concept that in rare cell detection there are events in normal healthy donors that mimic the immunophenotype of tumor cells.

As has been reviewed extensively elsewhere, there are many other technologies that are designed to increase the number of tumor cells that can be recovered from blood [51, 57]. The microfluidic CTC chips were designed to increment the interaction between capture antibodies and the cell and so improve recovery. While molecular evidence for tumor sampling was presented, the enumeration was not validated [58]. Indeed as for CellSearch, cells with matching immunophenotype to CTC were frequently described in normal donors [58–61].

Additional alternate approaches to rare cell enrichment used different characteristics of tumor cells as a means to distinguish them from normal blood cell populations. The methods of enrichment that replaced selection based on EpCAM include size selection using filters of various different designs [62–65], dielectrophoretic potential [66], microscopic characterization [67], inertial focusing, [68], and deformability [69], to name just a few. Many approaches have produced populations of cells that are unrelated to those identified by CellSearch and serve as useful discovery tools to advance the understanding of additional classes of rare cells in blood. In all examples, the effect of uncoupling from the validated enumeration approach includes a requirement to define the recovered cells by some method that presents an understanding of what the population represents.

Understanding these caveats, to what extent does the population of cells that are being enumerated as "CTC" beyond the CellSearch test include mutation-bearing bona fide tumor-derived cells? Legacy characterization of circulating epithelial cells identified aneusomy in recovered cells from adenocarcinoma of breast, lung, colon, prostate, and renal origin [45]. Numerous breast cancer studies have described a subpopulation of CTCs that over-express Her2 [43, 49, 70–72] demonstrating in parallel that all samples have mixed populations of Her2$^+$ and Her2$^-$ CTCs. In prostate cancer, there are CTCs that contain tumor-derived mutations reflecting genetic alterations in androgen receptor, TMPSSR and c-Myc locus [44, 61, 73–76]. In lung cancer, size-selected CTCs were shown to bear the *ALK* translocation in agreement with tissue biopsy analysis [77]. A molecular analysis of CTCs recovered by the CellSearch platform described an *EGFR* mutation within the EpCAM population in a fraction of preselected patients [48]. Using a CTC chip, Maheswaran et al. showed *EGFR* mutations in CTCs [78]. Other models where mutation-bearing CTC subpopulations have been described within the CTC pool include colorectal cancer [79] and malignant melanoma [46, 80]. Alternatively, the advent of accessible NGS platforms has allowed single-cell characterization of malignant populations of cells based on the detection of pathognomonic copy number variants (CNV) in many carcinoma models including prostate cancer and small-cell lung cancer [73, 81]. All of these detection tools emphasize that some but not all cells specifically enriched by any technology may be molecularly defined as a malignant tumor cell. Furthermore, capturing more cells by using either more antibodies or another physical property of the cell has only occasionally been demonstrated to result in increased capture of molecularly defined tumor cells [60, 82, 83].

Ultimately, there remains some misunderstanding about the proportion of CTCs that are mutation-bearing cells derived from a tumor, versus epithelial cells present either constitutively or due to inflammatory or healing mechanisms [52, 84]. All attempts to enumerate CTCs have revealed small numbers of circulating epithelial cells (CECs) in normal, healthy donors. Endogenous CECs are seen using emerging scanning platforms [85], expression analysis [86], and CTC chips in breast [41] or prostate cancer samples [76], or in lung cancer using high-definition imaging [87]. Without molecular classifiers, these CECs have been shown to contribute to an enumerated CTC population [52] even though they can also be shown to describe cells with a wild-type genomic configuration [79].

Boundaries Between Form and Function of Tumor Cells in Blood

In contrast to enumeration, the functional approach to identifying CTC relies on building protocols that support expansion of tumor cells in xenograft models or in vitro models. In building an understanding of which subset of cells in a tumor were capable of forming a tumor at a metastatic site, populations of tumor cells with different phenotypic characters were evaluated for their ability to form tumors in NOD/SCID immune-deficient animals. This approach led to the observation that as few as 100 tumor-derived cells with an immunophenotype that included expression of EpCAM could form a tumor in immune-deficient mice—the tumor-initiating cell (TIC). In contrast, 100-fold more cells recovered from a tumor that did not bear this phenotype were unsuccessful at supporting a xenograft tumor [37, 88]. Additional characterization of these cells defined a further distinct subpopulation that express aldehyde dehydrogenase (ALDH) expressed in the clinical samples associated with worse prognosis [89]. Indeed, these cells are capable of the epithelial to mesenchymal flexibility originally designed for organogenesis [38]. The emerging model suggests that epigenetic and genetic changes cause misregulation of this same organogenesis pathway enabling tumor cells with aberrant growth control to undergo a diseased version of this epithelial to mesenchymal transition, a process recognized as metastasis. Evidence for this relationship between the tumor-initiating cell and the stem cell can be seen in the related transcriptional programs exercised by the two populations [39].

Biologic data that supports this concept is seen in the parallels between the experiments that demonstrate metastatic potential in cells recovered from tumors and the related phenotype of those recovered from blood. EpCAM+/CD44+/CD24– cells are capable of forming tumors, as are EpCAM cells recovered from blood [90]. Indeed, by selecting EpCAM-expressing cells during metastatic stages of disease, it is possible to establish xenografts with as few as 50 cells [91]. In addition to being able to grow tumors directly, some CTCs may be cultured and maintain the same capacity to induce subsequent tumor formation in immune-deficient animals. Furthermore, the metastatic tropisms of these epithelial tumor cells recovered from blood are recapitulated in the xenograft model [92].

So, to what extent are the population of TIC and CTC overlapping? Both populations have been shown to include but are not limited to EpCAM-expressing cells. Cells with similar phenotypes from either the biopsy or the blood can form tumors in mice. Both populations are transcriptionally flexible and include expression fingerprints that indicate plasticity between epithelial and mesenchymal phenotypes [93]. Cells recovered from either compartment have shared mutations confirming both malignancy and a clearly demonstrated molecular relationship between the two [83, 94]. Finally, using a variety of tools to recover tumor cells from blood tissue, expression profiles that reflect the spectrum of epithelial to mesenchymal character have been described [41, 53, 95, 96]

These data start to define a spectrum of circulating tumor cell capabilities ranging from proliferative ALDH+ epithelial cells and more quiescent EMT like CD44+, CD24− cells. Included somewhere along this spectrum are the very same cells that have been prognostically enumerated by simple expression of cytokeratin (Fig. 7.1). This expression and functional spectrum aligns with the changing behavior of a population of tumor cells that leave a tumor site as part of the metastatic process. These are challenging models to dissect but the spectrum has been clearly demonstrated in in vivo tumor cell line models. The same cell populations can reduce their adhesive properties, thus inducing their release from the primary tumor site, but also can seed a remote site and support the proliferation necessary to drive metastasis [97]. In addition to a functional selection for cells with a regulated capacity to alternate between adherent and mobile, mechanical factors may also impact the

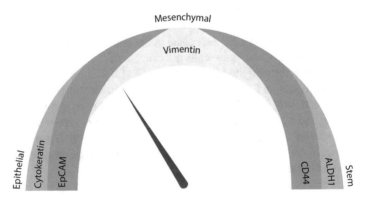

Fig. 7.1 The relationship between different categories of tumor-associated cells in circulation. Profiles and therefore function are determined by regulated expression of developmental gene programs. This figure includes representative classes and representative genes used to distinguish informative classes of cells

efficiency of this process. Clusters of tumor cells have been observed in blood in various models, both alone and with other classes of cells [61, 98]. In murine metastasis models, clusters of tumor cells were shown to be 23–50-fold more capable of forming metastatic events [99]. Transcriptional expression analysis did not identify significant differences in a clustered or single-cell event suggesting that it might be mechanical trapping of clusters that accounts for the association with metastases, a mechanical event that could start the extravasation process. However, clustering and indeed single cells are likely rapidly filtered from the blood as evidenced by the stark difference in CTC number between central and peripheral sources depending on the location of the tumor [100–104]. Therefore a greater understanding is clearly still required.

Functionally, the direction of these emerging data suggests that TIC and CTC models are starting to converge, as they should. This has a number of implications for molecular analysis of tumor cells recovered from blood. As the different populations of cells in blood acquire clearer definitions based on these functional and molecular descriptors, it increases the number of cells that may be interrogated. Of course, as soon as the population is changed, a new cell population ultimately has to be prospectively validated. However, by expanding the number of events that are molecularly informative, we increase the amount of information that may be gleaned from the cell populations in a liquid biopsy.

Circulating Tumor DNA

In contrast to the complexity of the cell populations, ctDNA in many ways provides a much simpler story. The presence of free nucleic acids in plasma was originally described over 50 years ago [105]. Largely due to the limits of technology, the field was initially focused on quantitation showing that a greater quantity of cell-free circulating DNA (ccfDNA) could be recovered from some cancer patients than normal healthy donors [106]. Subsequently, the tumor origin of that DNA was established [107]. Typically ccfDNA can be recovered in quantities ranging between 1 and 100 ng/mL. This constitutes several thousand genome equivalents, although it is to an important degree dependent on the extraction technology that is used [108]. Furthermore, the DNA recovered is generally all fragmented. The fragmentation patterns represent the apoptotic and necrotic biological processes that produce the DNA in the first place [109]. Consistent with this, the majority of the fragments correspond to the 162 base pair size associated with the nucleosome [110]. Therefore the ccfDNA compartment in plasma really represents a catabolite, a product of a largely normal process of eliminating unnecessary or damaged cells. The released ccfDNA has a short half-life, on the order of minutes, and is derived from any and all populations undergoing apoptosis or necrosis.

Although increasingly tools are being developed to detect cancer-derived ccfDNA, the baseline of ccfDNA in healthy donors and the majority of cancer samples are derived from the bone marrow [111]. This establishes a background ccfDNA population within which tumor-derived DNA has to be distinguished. This background drives sensitivity and specificity requirements for detection of ccfDNA that is tumor derived so that it remains possible to detect the very rare tumor fractions in the background of normal DNA [112].

The subpopulation of ccfDNA that is tumor derived is typically referred to as circulating tumor DNA (ctDNA). This tumor template is similarly fragmented and derives from all different sites of the tumor. As such, our understanding of the biological source of this material is still evolving. On balance, the data suggest that ctDNA is produced by an admixture of apoptosis and necrosis depending on stage, perfusion, and inherent cell turnover factors [113]. Generally, it is therefore thought to reflect the overall tumor burden which in turn is related to stage [114]. However there remains significant patient-to-patient variance and interventions such as chemotherapy and surgery can significantly alter ctDNA levels [113, 115–117]. In addition, the location of the tumor does seem to impact the quantity of recoverable ctDNA. This effect of location is obvious in the case of neurological tumors that are behind the blood–brain barrier. The variables that affect ctDNA prevalence in adenocarcinoma are less obvious and might be related to circulation, relationship between the cancer and the peripheral sample site, and half-life of the template [118].

ctDNA Boundaries Determined by Detection Tools

A second and important confounding factor is the challenge of distinguishing ctDNA from false-positive machine noise and from a category of biological noise that is only becoming apparent with the advent of next-generation sequencing.

The value of ctDNA is that it allows detection of changes in DNA sequence that can always be associated with transformation: Mutations alter growth by virtue of constitutively activating an oncogene or related gene product. Due to the clonal nature of cancer, daughter cells in a tumor will continue to reflect the same alteration and this will, with sufficient tumor burden, allow release of detectable numbers of mutated DNA molecules. One important aspect of detecting ctDNA has been the increased sensitivity of emerging molecular tools. The development of digital PCR [119] and next-generation sequencing tools [120] has allowed quantitative access to these molecules. Second, the information that can be gathered is a reflection of the classes of changes that are being measured as well as the signal to noise. So single-point variants (SNV) offer a highly specific and sensitive detection tool that has been evaluated using allele-specific PCR, digital PCR, and NGS.

Typically PCR-based technologies are focused on the specific site being evaluated. Sequencing in contrast will interrogate more extended sequences. As a result, a variety of technical modifications have been developed to provide increased sensitivity due to the contribution of both platform noise and biological noise that challenge detection at the very low sensitivities required. These techniques are typically focused on molecular barcoding to enable tracking of the source of the mutation.

This is needed to distinguish if an observed mutation is from the original template or introduced by the amplification process during the library assembly [114, 120–122]. Informatics tools can also help to align sequences that come from disparate parts of the genome (as occurs in rearrangements) and distinguish alterations that can be detected in normal healthy donors [123]. Together these approaches have shown that it is possible to identify SNV, translocations, and copy number variation in ccfDNA template. Tools are being developed and tested in a clinical setting now for specific clinical questions [119]. The success of this template has already been amply demonstrated with the rapid uptake of NIPT testing for suitable genomic alterations.

Despite these capabilities, the majority of cancer samples across all diseases present with fewer than 100 mutated DNA molecules in a standard blood sample, although this is elevated in later stage disease when the disease burden is greater [118]. Therefore there will remain biological thresholds to the limits of detection for ccfDNA fragments. Thus, we are no longer limited by our ability to detect mutated DNA events. Rather, the amount of tumor-derived material, volume of plasma necessary, and depth of sequencing required are becoming limiting [124]. Additionally, the biological process that results in ctDNA release is not well understood yet. The analysis of multiple metastatic sites in different cancers describes examples showing a very broad spectrum of heterogeneity in different diseases [15, 125, 126]. It is not yet clear whether the mechanisms of ctDNA release are equivalent at different metastatic sites. So how is this tumor heterogeneity manifest in the ctDNA template? This is in stark contrast to the biological selection associated with the presence of CTC and therefore ctcDNA in blood. The events that lead to ctDNA presence in plasma will cause molecular alterations to be detectable based on a selection process that may not be directly linked to the tumor clones that are driving disease. Conversely, by sampling the entire tumor, changes in molecular profile in response to treatment may prove to be predictive of response or resistance.

Finally, we must consider the informatics challenge of teasing apart signal from noise in a catabolite. If we restrict our analysis to well-defined cancer mutations such as *V600E BRAF* for instance, the risk of false-positive signal is calculable based on sequencing errors and template performance. Once we open the template to any mutation, the risks are more complicated. By restricting ourselves to mutations that are commonly associated with aberrant growth, we limit the degrees of freedom and reduce the informatics challenge of distinguishing signal from noise. The reason for this caution is related to the inevitable accumulation of damage in our DNA [127]. This damage is manifest because of accumulations of errors during the reproduction of cells to produce all the cells in an adult [128, 129]. In addition, as humans age, they accumulate clear evidence of damage [130]. The processes that spark tumorigenesis are not specific. So many changes occur due to exposures to carcinogens or UV light, for example, that do not always result in frank transformation but in a damaged cell that elevates the risk of cancer [131]. These events are certainly more prevalent in older individuals [132]. These hallmarks may be manifest in the ccfDNA compartment and do not necessarily presage the onset of frank tumorigenesis. Therefore, the applications of ccfDNA for targeted drug selection, minimal disease monitoring of known mutations, or cancer screening will require significantly more data to distinguish the source and implications of altered DNA sequence in the ccfDNA compartment.

Tying Two Tales Together

The excitement and interest in liquid biopsy are driven in large part by the ease of access to this tumor template and by the entirely new classes of information that are accessible. In many ways, it opens oncology up to the type of monitoring familiar in the infectious disease setting where emerging viral subtypes are monitored for emergence of drug resistance as well as pathogen fitness [133]. While more complex, monitoring capabilities are clearly needed in the treatment of cancer, these novel biomarkers have quickly become valued analytes. More than any other feature, the difference in sampling mechanism is the most profound difference between the gold standard biopsy tissue- and liquid biopsy-derived templates (Fig. 7.2). Whether it is ccfDNA or ctcDNA, blood-derived templates are derived from very rare events whether they are analyzed with different [115] or related technologies [134]. The applications therefore emerge from a clear understanding of the biological limitations of each biomarker as well as the classes of information that are valuable in a given clinical setting. BRAF V600 mutation status or EGFR T790M resistance mutation is very tractable in the ctDNA setting. However, splice variants such as AR-V7 or fusion targets such as ALK are much more tractable in cell-derived samples. In addition, the fact that all these templates are rare suggests that

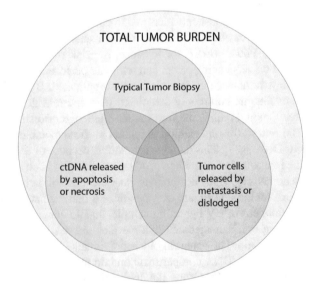

Fig. 7.2 Tumor biomarkers in blood are derived from any part of the parent tumor. Therefore ctDNA and circulating tumor cells must represent a subset of the parent. The overlaps are defined by the different mechanisms that produce each biomarker as well as the restrictions in the classes of biomarkers that can be detected. Similar to blood-derived biomarkers, the tumor biopsy also represents a subset of the total tumor burden and the typical biopsy is a small sample of the total disease

generating signal in either template is valuable. Data examining biomarkers that are compatible with both ctcDNA and cfDNA demonstrates that the different biological sampling manifest in ctDNA and ctcDNA does indeed produce complementary information in the two compartments [83]. This complementarity extends from the sampling methods to the biomarkers that can be analyzed, and to the biology that causes the different tumor templates to be present in blood in the first place. Ultimately, from the biology will come the application.

References

1. Vogelstein B, Kinzler KW (2004) Cancer genes and the pathways they control. Nat Med 10:789–799. doi:10.1038/nm1087
2. Hanahan D, Weinberg RA (2011) Hallmarks of cancer: the next generation. Cell 144:646–674. doi:10.1016/j.cell.2011.02.013
3. Dahabreh IJ, Linardou H, Siannis F et al (2008) Trastuzumab in the adjuvant treatment of early-stage breast cancer: a systematic review and meta-analysis of randomized controlled trials. Oncologist 13:620–630. doi:10.1634/theoncologist.2008-0001
4. Jabbour E, Lipton JH (2013) A critical review of trials of first-line BCR-ABL inhibitor treatment in patients with newly diagnosed chronic myeloid leukemia in chronic phase. Clin Lymphoma Myeloma Leuk 13:646–656. doi:10.1016/j.clml.2013.05.012
5. Klein CA (2013) Selection and adaptation during metastatic cancer progression. Nature 501:365–372. doi:10.1038/nature12628
6. Schmidt-Kittler O, Ragg T, Daskalakis A et al (2003) From latent disseminated cells to overt metastasis: genetic analysis of systemic breast cancer progression. Proc Natl Acad Sci U S A 100:7737–7742. doi:10.1073/pnas.1331931100
7. Bidard F-C, Peeters DJ, Fehm T et al (2014) Clinical validity of circulating tumour cells in patients with metastatic breast cancer: a pooled analysis of individual patient data. Lancet Oncol 15:406–414. doi:10.1016/S1470-2045(14)70069-5
8. Janni W, Rack B, Terstappen LW et al (2016) Pooled analysis of the prognostic relevance of circulating tumor cells in primary breast cancer. Clin Cancer Res 22:1–41. doi:10.1158/1078-0432.CCR-15-1603
9. Diaz LA, Bardelli A (2014) Liquid biopsies: genotyping circulating tumor DNA. J Clin Oncol Off J Am Soc Clin Oncol 32:579–586. doi:10.1200/JCO.2012.45.2011
10. Loman NJ, Misra RV, Dallman TJ et al (2012) Performance comparison of benchtop high-throughput sequencing platforms. Nat Biotechnol. doi:10.1038/nbt.2198
11. Banerji S, Cibulskis K, Rangel-Escareno C et al (2012) Sequence analysis of mutations and translocations across breast cancer subtypes. Nature 486:405–409. doi:10.1038/nature11154
12. Cancer Genome Atlas Network (2012) Comprehensive molecular portraits of human breast tumours. Nature 490:61–70. doi:10.1038/nature11412
13. Curtis C, Shah SP, Chin S-F et al (2012) The genomic and transcriptomic architecture of 2,000 breast tumours reveals novel subgroups. Nature 486:346–352. doi:10.1038/nature10983
14. Eirew P, Steif A, Khattra J et al (2014) Dynamics of genomic clones in breast cancer patient xenografts at single-cell resolution. Nature 518:422–426. doi:10.1038/nature13952
15. Gundem G, Van Loo P, Kremeyer B et al (2015) The evolutionary history of lethal metastatic prostate cancer. Nature 520:353–357. doi:10.1038/nature14347
16. Haber DA, Velculescu VE (2014) Blood-based analyses of cancer: circulating tumor cells and circulating tumor DNA. Cancer Discov 4:650–661. doi:10.1158/2159-8290.CD-13-1014
17. Ashworth TR (1869) A case of cancer in which cells similar to those in the tumours were seen in the blood after death. Aust Med J 14:146–147

18. Pantel K, Brakenhoff RH, Brandt B (2008a) Detection, clinical relevance and specific biological properties of disseminating tumour cells. Nat Rev Cancer 8:329–340. doi:10.1038/nrc2375
19. Gross HJ, Verwer B, Houck D et al (1995) Model study detecting breast cancer cells in peripheral blood mononuclear cells at frequencies as low as 10(−7). Proc Natl Acad Sci U S A 92:537–541
20. Racila E, Euhus D, Weiss AJ et al (1998) Detection and characterization of carcinoma cells in the blood. Proc Natl Acad Sci U S A 95:4589–4594
21. Vogel I, Krüger U, Marxsen J et al (1999) Disseminated tumor cells in pancreatic cancer patients detected by immunocytology: a new prognostic factor. Clin Cancer Res 5:593–599
22. Hayes DF, Cristofanilli M, Budd GT et al (2006) Circulating tumor cells at each follow-up time point during therapy of metastatic breast cancer patients predict progression-free and overall survival. Clin Cancer Res 12:4218–4224. doi:10.1158/1078-0432.CCR-05-2821
23. Alix-Panabières C, Bartkowiak K, Pantel K (2016) Functional studies on circulating and disseminated tumor cells in carcinoma patients. Mol Oncol 10:443–449. doi:10.1016/j.molonc.2016.01.004
24. Magbanua MJM, Park JW (2014) Advances in genomic characterization of circulating tumor cells. Cancer Metastasis Rev 33:757–769. doi:10.1007/s10555-014-9503-7
25. Allard WJ, Matera J, Miller MC et al (2004) Tumor cells circulate in the peripheral blood of all major carcinomas but not in healthy subjects or patients with nonmalignant diseases. Clin Cancer Res 10:6897–6904. doi:10.1158/1078-0432.CCR-04-0378
26. Cristofanilli M, Budd GT, Ellis MJ et al (2004) Circulating tumor cells, disease progression, and survival in metastatic breast cancer. N Engl J Med 351:781–791. doi:10.1056/NEJMoa040766
27. Cristofanilli M, Hayes DF, Budd GT et al (2005) Circulating tumor cells: a novel prognostic factor for newly diagnosed metastatic breast cancer. J Clin Oncol Off J Am Soc Clin Oncol 23:1420–1430. doi:10.1200/JCO.2005.08.140
28. Giuliano M, Giordano A, Jackson S et al (2011) Circulating tumor cells as prognostic and predictive markers in metastatic breast cancer patients receiving first-line systemic treatment. Breast Cancer Res 13:R67. doi:10.1186/bcr2907
29. Hayes DF (2006) Circulating tumor cells at each follow-up time point during therapy of metastatic breast cancer patients predict progression-free and overall survival. Clin Cancer Res 12:4218–4224. doi:10.1158/1078-0432.CCR-05-2821
30. Lucci A, Hall CS, Lodhi AK et al (2012) Circulating tumour cells in non-metastatic breast cancer: a prospective study. Lancet Oncol 13:688–695. doi:10.1016/S1470-2045(12)70209-7
31. Giuliano M, Giordano A, Jackson SD et al (2014) Circulating tumor cells as early predictors of metastatic spread in breast cancer patients with limited metastatic dissemination. Breast Cancer Res 16:440–449
32. Cohen SJ, Alpaugh RK, Gross S et al (2006) Isolation and characterization of circulating tumor cells in patients with metastatic colorectal cancer. Clin Colorectal Cancer 6:125–132. doi:10.3816/CCC.2006.n.029
33. Cohen SJ, Punt CJA, Iannotti N et al (2008) Relationship of circulating tumor cells to tumor response, progression-free survival, and overall survival in patients with metastatic colorectal cancer. J Clin Oncol Off J Am Soc Clin Oncol 26:3213–3221. doi:10.1200/JCO.2007.15.8923
34. Danila DC, Heller G, Gignac GA et al (2007) Circulating tumor cell number and prognosis in progressive castration-resistant prostate cancer. Clin Cancer Res 13:7053–7058. doi:10.1158/1078-0432.CCR-07-1506
35. de Bono JS, Scher HI, Montgomery RB et al (2008) Circulating tumor cells predict survival benefit from treatment in metastatic castration-resistant prostate cancer. Clin Cancer Res 14:6302–6309. doi:10.1158/1078-0432.CCR-08-0872
36. Tsai JH, Donaher JL, Murphy DA et al (2012) Spatiotemporal regulation of epithelial-mesenchymal transition is essential for squamous cell carcinoma metastasis. Cancer Cell 22:725–736. doi:10.1016/j.ccr.2012.09.022

37. Al-Hajj M, Wicha MS, Benito-Hernandez A et al (2003) Prospective identification of tumorigenic breast cancer cells. Proc Natl Acad Sci U S A 100:3983–3988. doi:10.1073/pnas.0530291100
38. Liu S, Cong Y, Wang D et al (2014) Breast cancer stem cells transition between epithelial and mesenchymal states reflective of their normal counterparts. Stem Cell Reports 2:78–91. doi:10.1016/j.stemcr.2013.11.009
39. Ye X, Tam WL, Shibue T et al (2015) Distinct EMT programs control normal mammary stem cells and tumour-initiating cells. Nature 525:256–260. doi:10.1038/nature14897
40. Lecharpentier A, Vielh P, Perez-Moreno P et al (2011) Detection of circulating tumour cells with a hybrid (epithelial/mesenchymal) phenotype in patients with metastatic non-small cell lung cancer. Br J Cancer 105:1338–1341. doi:10.1038/bjc.2011.405
41. Yu M, Bardia A, Wittner BS et al (2013) Circulating breast tumor cells exhibit dynamic changes in epithelial and mesenchymal composition. Science 339:580–584. doi:10.1126/science.1228522
42. Mego M, Gao H, Lee B-N et al (2012) Prognostic value of EMT-circulating tumor cells in metastatic breast cancer patients undergoing high-dose chemotherapy with autologous hematopoietic stem cell transplantation. J Cancer 3:369–380. doi:10.7150/jca.5111
43. Meng S, Tripathy D, Shete S et al (2004) HER-2 gene amplification can be acquired as breast cancer progresses. Proc Natl Acad Sci U S A 101:9393–9398. doi:10.1073/pnas.0402993101
44. Leversha M, Han J, Asgari Z, Danila D (2009) Fluorescence in situ hybridization analysis of circulating tumor cells in metastatic prostate cancer. Clin Cancer Res 15(6):2091–2097
45. Fehm T, Sagalowsky A, Clifford E et al (2002) Cytogenetic evidence that circulating epithelial cells in patients with carcinoma are malignant. Clin Cancer Res 8:2073–2084
46. Ulmer A, Schmidt-Kittler O, Fischer J et al (2004) Immunomagnetic enrichment, genomic characterization, and prognostic impact of circulating melanoma cells. Clin Cancer Res 10:531–537
47. Flores LM, Kindelberger DW, Ligon AH et al (2010) Improving the yield of circulating tumour cells facilitates molecular characterisation and recognition of discordant HER2 amplification in breast cancer. Br J Cancer 102:1495–1502. doi:10.1038/sj.bjc.6605676
48. Punnoose EA, Atwal S, Liu W et al (2012) Evaluation of circulating tumor cells and circulating tumor DNA in non-small cell lung cancer: association with clinical endpoints in a phase II clinical trial of pertuzumab and erlotinib. Clin Cancer Res 18:2391–2401. doi:10.1158/1078-0432.CCR-11-3148
49. Punnoose EA, Atwal SK, Spoerke JM et al (2010) Molecular biomarker analyses using circulating tumor cells. PLoS One 5:e12517. doi:10.1371/journal.pone.0012517
50. Riethdorf S, Fritsche H, Müller V, Rau T (2007) Detection of circulating tumor cells in peripheral blood of patients with metastatic breast cancer: a validation study of the CellSearch system. Clin Cancer Res 13(3)
51. Parkinson DR, Dracopoli N, Petty BG et al (2012) Considerations in the development of circulating tumor cell technology for clinical use. J Transl Med 10:138. doi:10.1186/1479-5876-10-138
52. Pantel K, Denève E, Nocca D, Coffy A et al (2012) Circulating epithelial cells in patients with benign colon diseases. Clin Chem 58:936–940
53. Pecot CV, Bischoff FZ, Mayer JA et al (2011) A novel platform for detection of CK+ and CK− CTCs. Cancer Discov 1:580–586. doi:10.1158/2159-8290.CD-11-0215
54. Fehm T, Hoffmann O, Aktas B et al (2009) Detection and characterization of circulating tumor cells in blood of primary breast cancer patients by RT-PCR and comparison to status of bone marrow disseminated cells. Breast Cancer Res 11:R59. doi:10.1186/bcr2349
55. Müller V, Riethdorf S, Rack B et al (2013) Prognostic impact of circulating tumor cells assessed with the CellSearch SystemTM and AdnaTest BreastTM in metastatic breast cancer patients: the DETECT study. Breast Cancer Res 14:1–8
56. Aktas B, Müller V, Tewes M et al (2011) Gynecologic oncology. Gynecol Oncol 122:356–360. doi:10.1016/j.ygyno.2011.04.039
57. Friedlander TW, Premasekharan G, Paris PL (2014) Pharmacology & therapeutics. Pharmacol Ther:1–10. doi:10.1016/j.pharmthera.2013.12.011

58. Nagrath S, Sequist LV, Maheswaran S et al (2007) Isolation of rare circulating tumour cells in cancer patients by microchip technology. Nature 450:1235–1239. doi:10.1038/nature06385
59. Dickson M, Tsinberg P, Tang Z, Bischoff F (2011) Efficient capture of circulating tumor cells with a novel immunocytochemical microfluidic device. Biomicrofluidics 5(3):34119–3411915
60. Mayer JA, Pham T, Wong KL et al (2011) FISH-based determination of HER2 status in circulating tumor cells isolated with the microfluidic CEE! platform. Cancer Genet 204:589–595. doi:10.1016/j.cancergen.2011.10.011
61. Stott SL, Hsu C-H, Tsukrov DI et al (2010a) Isolation of circulating tumor cells using a microvortex-generating herringbone-chip. Proc Natl Acad Sci U S A 107:18392–18397. doi:10.1073/pnas.1012539107
62. Adams DL, Stefansson S, Haudenschild C et al (2014) Cytometric characterization of circulating tumor cells captured by microfiltration and their correlation to the Cellsearch ®CTC test. Cytometry A 87:137–144. doi:10.1002/cyto.a.22613
63. Coumans FAW, van Dalum G, Beck M, Terstappen LWMM (2013) Filter characteristics influencing circulating tumor cell enrichment from whole blood. PLoS One 8:e61770. doi:10.1371/journal.pone.0061770.t003
64. De Giorgi V, Pinzani P, Salvianti F et al (2010) Application of a filtration- and isolation-by-size technique for the detection of circulating tumor cells in cutaneous melanoma. J Invest Dermatol 130:2440–2447. doi:10.1038/jid.2010.141
65. Xu T, Lu B, Tai Y-C, Goldkorn A (2010) A cancer detection platform which measures telomerase activity from live circulating tumor cells captured on a microfilter. Cancer Res 70:6420–6426. doi:10.1158/0008-5472.CAN-10-0686
66. O'Shannessy D, Davis D, Anderes K, Somers E (2016) Isolation of circulating tumor cells from multiple epithelial cancers with apostream for detecting (or monitoring) the expression of folate receptor alpha. BMI:7–12. doi:10.4137/BMI.S35075
67. Werner SL, Graf RP, Landers M et al (2015) Analytical validation and capabilities of the epic CTC platform: enrichment-free circulating tumour cell detection and characterization. J Circ Biomark:1–13. doi:10.5772/60725
68. Ozkumur E, Shah AM, Ciciliano JC et al (2013) Inertial focusing for tumor antigen-dependent and -independent sorting of rare circulating tumor cells. Sci Transl Med 5 . doi:10.1126/scitranslmed.3005616179ra47–179ra47
69. Tse H, Gossett DR, Moon YS et al (2013) Quantitative diagnosis of malignant pleural effusions by single-cell mechanophenotyping. Sci Transl Med 5:1–9
70. Ignatiadis M, Rothé F, Chaboteaux C et al (2011) HER2-positive circulating tumor cells in breast cancer. PLoS One 6:e15624
71. Kim P, Liu X, Lee T et al (2011) Highly sensitive proximity mediated immunoassay reveals HER2 status conversion in the circulating tumor cells of metastatic breast cancer patients. Proteome Sci 9:75
72. Pestrin M, Bessi S, Puglisi F et al (2012) Final results of a multicenter phase II clinical trial evaluating the activity of single-agent lapatinib in patients with HER2-negative metastatic breast cancer and HER2-positive circulating tumor cells. A proof-of-concept study. Breast Cancer Res Treat 134:283–289. doi:10.1007/s10549-012-2045-1
73. Attard G, Swennenhuis JF, Olmos D et al (2009) Characterization of ERG, AR and PTEN gene status in circulating tumor cells from patients with castration-resistant prostate cancer. Cancer Res 69:2912–2918. doi:10.1158/0008-5472.CAN-08-3667
74. Danila DC, Anand A, Sung CC et al (2011) TMPRSS2-ERG status in circulating tumor cells as a predictive biomarker of sensitivity in castration-resistant prostate cancer patients treated with abiraterone acetate. Eur Urol 60:897–904. doi:10.1016/j.eururo.2011.07.011
75. Jiang Y, Palma JF, Agus DB et al (2010) Detection of androgen receptor mutations in circulating tumor cells in castration-resistant prostate cancer. Clin Chem 56:1492–1495. doi:10.1373/clinchem.2010.143297
76. Stott SL, Lee RJ, Nagrath S et al (2010b) Isolation and characterization of circulating tumor cells from patients with localized and metastatic prostate cancer. Sci Transl Med 2 . doi:10.1126/scitranslmed.300040325ra23

77. Ilie M, Long E, Butori C et al (2012) ALK-gene rearrangement: a comparative analysis on circulating tumour cells and tumour tissue from patients with lung adenocarcinoma. Ann Oncol. doi:10.1093/annonc/mds137

78. Maheswaran S, Sequist LV, Nagrath S et al (2008) Detection of mutations in EGFR in circulating lung-cancer cells. N Engl J Med 359:366–377

79. Heitzer E, Auer M, Gasch C et al (2013) Complex tumor genomes inferred from single circulating tumor cells by array-CGH and next-generation sequencing. Cancer Res 73:2965–2975. doi:10.1158/0008-5472.CAN-12-4140

80. Sakaizawa K, Goto Y, Kiniwa Y et al (2012) Mutation analysis of BRAF and KIT in circulating melanoma cells at the single cell level. Br J Cancer 106:939–946. doi:10.1038/bjc.2012.12

81. Hodgkinson CL, Morrow CJ, Li Y et al (2014) Tumorigenicity and genetic profiling of circulating tumor cells in small-cell lung cancer. Nat Med:1–9. doi:10.1038/nm.3600

82. Lynch TJ, Bell DW, Sordella R et al (2004) Activating mutations in the epidermal growth factor receptor underlying responsiveness of non-small-cell lung cancer to gefitinib. N Engl J Med 350:2129–2139. doi:10.1056/NEJMoa040938

83. Strauss WM, Carter C, SImmons J et al (2016) Analysis of tumor template from multiple compartments in a blood sample provides complementary access to peripheral tumor biomarkers. Oncotarget 7(18):26724–26738. doi:10.18632/oncotarget.8494

84. Hardingham JE, Hewett PJ, Sage RE et al (2000) Molecular detection of blood-borne epithelial cells in colorectal cancer patients and in patients with benign bowel disease. Int J Cancer 89:8–13

85. Zhao M, Schiro PG, Kuo JS et al (2013) An automated high-throughput counting method for screening circulating tumor cells in peripheral blood. Anal Chem 85(4):2465–2471. doi:10.1021/ac400193b

86. You F, Roberts LA, Kang SP et al (2008) Low-level expression of HER2 and CK19 in normal peripheral blood mononuclear cells: relevance for detection of circulating tumor cells. J Hematol Oncol 1:2. doi:10.1186/1756-8722-1-2

87. Nieva J, Wendel M, Luttgen MS et al (2012) High-definition imaging of circulating tumor cells and associated cellular events in non-small cell lung cancer patients: a longitudinal analysis. Phys Biol 9:016004. doi:10.1088/1478-3975/9/1/016004

88. Li C, Heidt DG, Dalerba P et al (2007) Identification of pancreatic cancer stem cells. Cancer Res 67:1030–1037. doi:10.1158/0008-5472.CAN-06-2030

89. Ginestier C, Hur MH, Charafe-Jauffret E et al (2007) ALDH1 is a marker of normal and malignant human mammary stem cells and a predictor of poor clinical outcome. Cell Stem Cell 1:555–567. doi:10.1016/j.stem.2007.08.014

90. Baccelli I, Schneeweiss A, Riethdorf S et al (2013) Identification of a population of blood circulating tumor cells from breast cancer patients that initiates metastasis in a xenograft assay. Nat Biotechnol:1–7. doi:10.1038/nbt.2576

91. Rossi E, Rugge M, Facchinetti A et al (2014) Retaining the long-survive capacity of Circulating Tumor Cells (CTCs) followed by xeno-transplantation: not only from metastatic cancer of the breast but also of prostate cancer patients. Oncoscience 1:49–56

92. Zhang L, Ridgway LD, Wetzel MD et al (2013) The identification and characterization of breast cancer CTCs competent for brain metastasis. Sci Transl Med 5 . doi:10.1126/scitranslmed.3005109180ra48

93. Yu M, Stott S, Toner M et al (2011) Circulating tumor cells: approaches to isolation and characterization. J Cell Biol 192:373–382. doi:10.1083/jcb.201010021

94. Zhang Z, Shiratsuchi H, Lin J et al (2014) Expansion of CTCs from early stage lung cancer patients using a microfluidic co-culture model. Oncotarget 5(23):12383–12397

95. Chen C-L, Mahalingam D, Osmulski P et al (2012) Single-cell analysis of circulating tumor cells identifies cumulative expression patterns of EMT-related genes in metastatic prostate cancer. Prostate. doi:10.1002/pros.22625

96. Krebs MG, Hou J-M, Sloane R et al (2012) Analysis of circulating tumor cells in patients with non-small cell lung cancer using epithelial marker-dependent and -independent approaches. J Thorac Oncol 7:306–315. doi:10.1097/JTO.0b013e31823c5c16

97. Celià-Terrassa T, Meca-Cortés Ó, Mateo F et al (2012) Epithelial-mesenchymal transition can suppress major attributes of human epithelial tumor-initiating cells. J Clin Invest 122:1849–1868. doi:10.1172/JCI59218

98. Hou J-M, Krebs MG, Lancashire L et al (2012) Clinical significance and molecular characteristics of circulating tumor cells and circulating tumor microemboli in patients with small-cell lung cancer. J Clin Oncol Off J Am Soc Clin Oncol. doi:10.1200/JCO.2010.33.3716

99. Aceto N, Bardia A, Miyamoto DT et al (2014) Circulating tumor cell clusters are oligoclonal precursors of breast cancer metastasis. Cell 158:1110–1122. doi:10.1016/j.cell.2014.07.013

100. Hashimoto M, Tanaka F, Yoneda K et al (2014) Significant increase in circulating tumour cells in pulmonary venous blood during surgical manipulation in patients with primary lung cancer. Interact Cardiovasc Thorac Surg 18:775–783. doi:10.1093/icvts/ivu048

101. Okumura Y, Tanaka F, Yoneda K et al (2009) Circulating tumor cells in pulmonary venous blood of primary lung cancer patients. Ann Thorac Surg 87:1669–1675. doi:10.1016/j.athoracsur.2009.03.073

102. Peeters DJE, Brouwer A, Van den Eynden GG et al (2015) Circulating tumour cells and lung microvascular tumour cell retention in patients with metastatic breast and cervical cancer. Cancer Lett 356:872–879. doi:10.1016/j.canlet.2014.10.039

103. Reddy RM, Murlidhar V, Zhao L et al (2016) Pulmonary venous blood sampling significantly increases the yield of circulating tumor cells in early-stage lung cancer. J Thorac Cardiovasc Surg 151:852–858. doi:10.1016/j.jtcvs.2015.09.126

104. Terai M, Mu Z, Eschelman DJ et al (2015) Arterial blood, rather than venous blood, is a better source for circulating melanoma cells. EBioMedicine 2(11):1821–1826. doi:10.1016/j.ebiom.2015.09.019

105. Mandel P (1948) Les acides nucleiques du plasma sanguin chez l'homme. CR Acad Sci Paris 142:241–243

106. Stroun M, Anker P, Lyautey J et al (1987) Isolation and characterization of DNA from the plasma of cancer patients. Eur J Cancer Clin Oncol 23:707–712

107. Stroun M, Anker P, Maurice P et al (1989) Neoplastic characteristics of the DNA found in the plasma of cancer patients. Oncology 46:318–322

108. Devonshire AS, Whale AS, Gutteridge A et al (2014) Towards standardisation of cell-free DNA measurement in plasma: controls for extraction efficiency, fragment size bias and quantification. Anal Bioanal Chem 406:6499–6512. doi:10.1007/s00216-014-7835-3

109. Jahr S, Hentze H, Englisch S et al (2001) DNA fragments in the blood plasma of cancer patients: quantitations and evidence for their origin from apoptotic and necrotic cells. Cancer Res 61:1659–1665

110. Fan HC, Blumenfeld YJ, Chitkara U et al (2010) Analysis of the size distributions of fetal and maternal cell-free DNA by paired-end sequencing. Clin Chem 56:1279–1286. doi:10.1373/clinchem.2010.144188

111. Lui YYN, Chik K-W, Chiu RWK et al (2002) Predominant hematopoietic origin of cell-free DNA in plasma and serum after sex-mismatched bone marrow transplantation. Clin Chem 48:421–427

112. Engelman JA, Mukohara T, Zejnullahu K et al (2006) Allelic dilution obscures detection of a biologically significant resistance mutation in EGFR-amplified lung cancer. J Clin Invest 116:2695–2706. doi:10.1172/JCI28656

113. Diehl F, Schmidt K, Choti MA et al (2008) Circulating mutant DNA to assess tumor dynamics. Nat Med 14:985–990. doi:10.1038/nm.1789

114. Forshew T, Murtaza M, Parkinson C et al (2012) Noninvasive identification and monitoring of cancer mutations by targeted deep sequencing of plasma DNA. Sci Transl Med 4:136ra68. doi:10.1126/scitranslmed.3003726

115. Dawson S-J, Tsui DWY, Murtaza M et al (2013) Analysis of circulating tumor DNA to monitor metastatic breast cancer. N Engl J Med 368:1199–1209. doi:10.1056/NEJMoa1213261

116. Hamakawa T, Kukita Y, Kurokawa Y et al (2014) Monitoring gastric cancer progression with circulating tumour DNA. Br J Cancer 112:352–356. doi:10.1038/bjc.2014.609

117. Lipson EJ, Velculescu VE, Pritchard TS et al (2014) Circulating tumor DNA analysis as a real-time method for monitoring tumor burden in melanoma patients undergoing treatment with immune checkpoint blockade. J Immunother Cancer 2:42. doi:10.1186/s40425-014-0042-0

118. Bettegowda C, Sausen M, Leary RJ et al (2014) Detection of circulating tumor DNA in early- and late-stage human malignancies. Sci Transl Med 6 . doi:10.1126/scitranslmed.3007094224ra24–224ra24

119. Sacher AG, Paweletz C, Dahlberg SE et al (2016) Prospective validation of rapid plasma genotyping for the detection of EGFR and KRAS mutations in advanced lung cancer. JAMA Oncol 2(8):1014–1022. doi:10.1001/jamaoncol.2016.0173

120. Lanman RB, Mortimer SA, Zill OA et al (2015) Analytical and clinical validation of a digital sequencing panel for quantitative, highly accurate evaluation of cell-free circulating tumor DNA. PLoS One 10:e0140712

121. Kinde I, Wu J, Papadopoulos N et al (2011) Detection and quantification of rare mutations with massively parallel sequencing. Proc Natl Acad Sci U S A 108:9530–9535. doi:10.1073/pnas.1105422108

122. Newman AM, Bratman SV, To J et al (2014) An ultrasensitive method for quantitating circulating tumor DNA with broad patient coverage. Nat Med 20:548–554. doi:10.1038/nm.3519

123. Leary RJ, Sausen M, Kinde I et al (2012) Detection of chromosomal alterations in the circulation of cancer patients with whole-genome sequencing. Sci Transl Med 4:162ra154–162ra154. doi:10.1126/scitranslmed.3004742

124. Newman AM, Lovejoy AF, Klass DM et al (2016) Integrated digital error suppression for improved detection of circulating tumor DNA. Nat Biotechnol. doi:10.1038/nbt.3520

125. Fujimoto J, Wedge DC, Song X et al (2014) Intratumor heterogeneity in localized lung adenocarcinomas delineated by multiregion sequencing. Science 346:256–259. doi:10.1126/science.1256930

126. Gerlinger M, Rowan AJ, Horswell S et al (2012) Intratumor heterogeneity and branched evolution revealed by multiregion sequencing. N Engl J Med 366:883–892. doi:10.1056/NEJMoa1113205

127. Vijg J (2014) Somatic mutations, genome mosaicism, cancer and aging. Curr Opin Genet Dev 26:141–149. doi:10.1016/j.gde.2014.04.002

128. Behjati S, Huch M, van Boxtel R et al (2014) Genome sequencing of normal cells reveals developmental lineages and mutational processes. Nature 513:422–425. doi:10.1038/nature13448

129. Tomasetti C, Vogelstein B (2015) Variation in cancer risk among tissues can be explained by the number of stem cell divisions. Science 347:78–81. doi:10.1073/pnas.1221724110

130. Soares JP, Cortinhas A, Bento T, Leitão JC (2014) Aging and DNA damage in humans: a meta-analysis study. Aging (Albany NY) 6(6):432–439

131. Genovese G, Kähler AK, Handsaker RE et al (2014) Clonal hematopoiesis and blood-cancer risk inferred from blood DNA sequence. N Engl J Med 371:2477–2487. doi:10.1056/NEJMoa1409405

132. Laurie CC, Laurie CA, Rice K et al (2012) Detectable clonal mosaicism from birth to old age and its relationship to cancer. Nat Genet 44:642–650. doi:10.1038/ng.2271

133. Iyidogan P, Anderson K (2014) Current perspectives on HIV-1 antiretroviral drug resistance. Viruses 6:4095–4139. doi:10.3390/v6104095

134. Rothwell DG, Smith N, Morris D et al (2016) Genetic profiling of tumours using both circulating free DNA and circulating tumour cells isolated from the same preserved whole blood sample. Mol Oncol 10:566–574. doi:10.1016/j.molonc.2015.11.006

Chapter 8
Exosomes: The Next Small Thing

Vincent J. O'Neill

Abstract Exosomes are a class of microvesicles that function as intercellular signalers in both healthy and disease states. Thought initially to be simply cellular debris, exosomes have been known about for close to 30 years, but only recently has their crucial physiological function begun to be elucidated. Their presence in most biofluids (including blood, urine, and sputum) offers significant potential for diagnostic and therapeutic applications.

Keywords Exosomes • Microvesicles • microRNA • Liquid biopsy • RNA therapeutics

Introduction

Intercellular communication is a fundamental hallmark of multicellular organisms, and may be mediated by direct cellular contact (via surface proteins) or by interaction with secreted molecules (e.g., growth factors, hormones). A large body of evidence now establishes a third method of cellular communication, facilitated by extracellular vesicles (EVs), including exosomes. These structures are highly complex, containing several classes of macromolecules, and have been shown to be involved in physiologic and pathophysiologic conditions, including cancer, immune processes, and inflammation to name only a few. As discussed below, the ability afforded by these vesicles to provide a comprehensive snapshot of cellular processes offers great promise in the area of noninvasive diagnostics. Further, their potential as delivery systems for therapeutic payloads has begun to be explored.

V.J. O'Neill (✉)
Mirna Therapeutics, 2150 Woodward Street, Suite 100, Austin, TX 78744, USA
e-mail: voneill@mirnarx.com

© Springer International Publishing AG 2017
M. Cristofanilli (ed.), *Liquid Biopsies in Solid Tumors*, Cancer Drug Discovery and Development, DOI 10.1007/978-3-319-50956-3_8

Discovery

Exosomes were first described in the mid-1980s by Johnson and colleagues, who found that, in maturing mammalian reticulocytes, the transferrin receptor and some other membrane-associated elements are selectively released in multivesicular body- (MVB-) derived circulating vesicles, which they named exosomes [1, 2]. One of the first lines of evidence that tumor cells shed membrane vesicles was however provided much earlier, when Friend and coworkers in the late 1970s described them as *"rare, pleomorphic membrane-lined particles ranging broadly in size between 400 and 1200 Å,"* in cell lines derived from patients with Hodgkin's disease [3]. A year later an independent study identified plasma-derived vesicles released by murine leukemia cells [4]. Despite these important advances, the general assumption remained that these vesicles represented cell debris, and were of limited interest. This position was revised after the discovery that extracellular vesicles contain RNA as well as proteins, and that the vesicular content was not random, but specifically packaged by an active cellular process. Today, exosome and microvesicle research is an area of intense interest. A literature search via PubMed in 2016 returns in excess of 2000 citations, underscoring the interest in the field.

Genesis

Microvesicles (MVs) are a heterogeneous group of extracellular bodies, encompassing particles from 30 nm to a few microns in size. In response to ongoing debate on classification and nomenclature, a number of systems have been proposed. A broadly accepted method of classifying MVs is based primarily on size (and secondarily on protein content): the largest, apoptotic bodies, range from 1 to 5 μm; next, microvesicles have a size range from 1 μm to 100 nm; and lastly, the smallest MVs, exosomes, have a size range of 30–100 nm. It is now generally recognized however that size and protein composition alone are not enough to classify MVs, and that mode of production is more informative. In order therefore to be considered an exosome, an MV has to be formed by invagination of a multivesicular body (MVB), a specialized endosome, which then fuses with the cell membrane.

Aside from size, exosomes have a characteristic density which can be exploited in their isolation. Additionally, they seem to share specific surface proteins—independent of cell of origin—which identifies them, and may be exploited in their isolation and characterization. Specifically, because of their cellular origin, exosomes bear specific protein markers of the endosomal pathway, such as tetraspanins (CD63, CD9, and CD81), heat-shock proteins (HSP70), and proteins from the Rab family, Tsg101 and Alix, which are not found in other types of vesicles of similar size.

As might be surmised from their content, exosome formation is a highly regulated process which includes four stages: initiation, endocytosis, MVB formation,

Fig. 8.1 Biogenesis of exosomes. Reprinted from Hu et al. with permission of the publisher. Copyright © 2012, Frontiers in Genetics

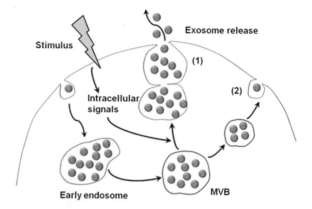

and exosome secretion [5]. Multivesicular bodies are endocytic structures formed by the budding of an endosomal membrane into the lumen of the compartment. After vesicular accumulation, the MVBs are either sorted for cargo degradation in the lysosome or released into the extracellular space as exosomes by fusing with the plasma membrane (Fig. 8.1).

It is obvious from the foregoing that the biogenesis of exosomes requires cellular expenditure of energy and resources, implying crucial functional importance for exosomes.

Structure and Content

Exosomes are surrounded by a lipid bilayer which confers considerable stability to their contents. It has been demonstrated that they are stable across freeze-thaw cycles, and temperature variations [6], making them ideal for diagnostic applications (see below). The lipid composition has also been suggested to be functionally relevant: several reports have suggested that phosphatidylserine [7] and prostaglandins [8] may play an important role in exosomal functions.

A major breakthrough in exosome research came with the demonstration in 2007 that not only they contain nucleic acid, predominantly RNA, but also these could be transferred between cells [9], fundamentally changing the view of exosomes as mere cellular detritus. Microarray assessments revealed the presence of RNA from approximately 1300 genes, many of which are not present in the cytoplasm of the donor cell, and that these RNAs (mRNA and miRNA) were functional. The authors coined the term "exosomal shuttle RNA" (esRNA) for this RNA, based on their findings. Later studies reported on the RNA contents of EV isolates from other cell cultures [10] and from various body fluids [11–14]. Indeed, hematopoietic cells (B cells, T cells, dendritic cells, mast cells, and platelets), intestinal epithelial cells, Schwann cells, neuronal cells, adipocytes, fibroblasts (NIH3T3), and tumor cells have all been shown to secrete MVB internal vesicles [15] (Fig. 8.2).

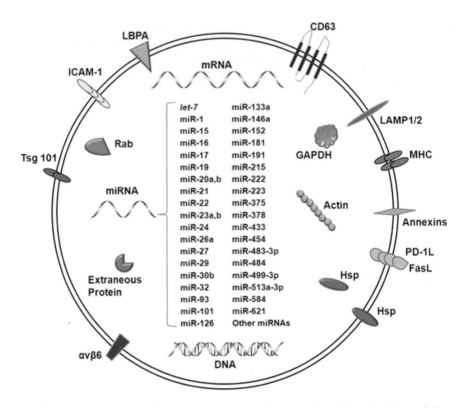

Fig. 8.2 Major classes of molecules within exosomes. Reprinted from Hu et al. with permission of the publisher. Copyright © 2012, Frontiers in Genetics

According to ExoCarta, a useful and comprehensive exosome content database, 4563 proteins, 194 lipids, 1639 mRNAs, and 764 miRNAs have been identified in exosomes from multiple organisms [16]. They therefore contain all the macromolecules that might be of interest from a diagnostic viewpoint. Specific exosomal cargoes are discussed below.

MicroRNAs

MicroRNAs (miRNAs) are small noncoding, naturally occurring RNA molecules that posttranscriptionally modulate gene expression and determine cell fate by regulating multiple gene products and cellular pathways [17]. The misregulation of miRNAs is often a serious detrimental cellular event that can contribute to the development of human disease including cancer [18, 19]. miRNAs deregulated in cancer target multiple oncogenic signaling pathways and have therefore the potential of becoming powerful therapeutic agents [20, 21].

It has now been established that there are two mechanisms whereby miRNA avoids RNA-ase-mediated degradation: by encapsulation in exosomes, and by association with AGO proteins. In fact, the majority of miRNAs in the circulation appear to be AGO bound; however specific sorting and packaging of miRNAs into exosomes make the vesicle-bound fraction especially interesting.

The discovery of miRNAs adds another layer of gene regulation that is subject to change in human disease including cancer. Similar to protein-encoding genes, miRNAs are now supported by expression data and experimental evidence in vitro and in vivo that marks these interesting RNA molecules as promising therapeutic targets: miRNAs frequently acquire a gain or a loss of function in cancer; and miRNAs play a causative role in the development of cancer [19].

mRNA

Exosomes are also known to contain mRNA although these species of RNA appear to be found at lower abundance compared to the small RNA components [22]. Hong et al. profiled the mRNA of exosomes derived from a colorectal cancer cell line, identifying over 11,000 distinct mRNA molecules within the exosome samples [23]. The authors point out that many of these mRNAs are involved in cellular processes such as cell division, cell cycle, and chromosome segregation. Similar mRNA profiling was completed for exosomes derived from samples derived from patients with glioblastoma [24]. Importantly, mRNA for a mutant version of EGFR (EGFRvIII) was identified by these researchers in exosomes isolated from the plasma of some patients (7 out of 25). The discovery of mRNA encoding a mutant protein in circulating exosomes has significant implications for their use in noninvasive diagnosis, as discussed in detail below.

Proteins

The proteins most frequently identified in exosomes are membrane transporters and fusion proteins (e.g., GTPases, annexins, and flotillin), heat-shock proteins (e.g., HSC70), tetraspanins (e.g., CD9, CD63, and CD81), MVB biogenesis proteins (e.g., alix and TSG101), and lipid-related proteins and phospholipases [25, 26]. Several proteins are recognized as specific exosomal markers, among which the tetraspanins, CD63 and CD81, are the most commonly used.

The list of proteins found in exosomes continues to expand, as can be seen by referencing ExoCarta [16]. Oncogenes that are associated with various types of cancer are frequently found in the exosomes secreted by tumor cells. For example, full-length EGFR has been identified in exosomes isolated from pancreatic cell lines [27]. Given the abundance of exosomes in urine, and the ease with which they can be isolated from this medium, a considerable body of evidence has accumulated on the protein content of urinary exosomes, both within urogenital and systemic conditions [28, 29]. Many of these data are collated on the Urinary Exosome Protein Database, an online resource curated by the National Heart Lung and Blood Institute [30].

Lipids

Several reports have suggested that certain lipid components of exosomes, such as phosphatidylserine [16] and prostaglandins [17], may play an important role in exosomal functions. Interestingly, the content of lipids in exosomes differs substantially from that of the parental cells. While the content of sphingomyelin, phosphatidylserine, phosphatidylinositol, ceramides, and cholesterol is highly increased in exosomes, the content of phosphatidylcholine is typically decreased. [31, 32]. Presence of phosphatidylserine on the outer membrane of exosomes can function in exosome recognition and internalization by recipient cells [33] and therefore exosomes may function as lipid carriers.

A crucial concept that will be clear from the foregoing is *cargo sorting*, i.e., the RNA within exosomes is specific and not the result of random sampling of cytosol content. The importance of this is discussed in detail below.

Function

As will be clear from the foregoing, the major role of exosomes seems to be the transport of bioactive molecules between cells, such as mRNA and miRNA, with consequences in targeted cell phenotypes. The functional relevance of exosomes, with a particular emphasis on cancer, will now be discussed.

Exosomes in Cancer: Angiogenesis, Immunity, and Metastasis

Tumor-derived exosomes can now be isolated from tumors and bodily fluids from patients with tumors with relative ease. Since cancer-derived exosomes carry both genomic and proteomic material, as detailed above, and can transfer information at a distance, it makes sense that they play a role in the varied mechanisms malignant cells utilize in their growth and metastasis. For instance, the protein *EGFRvIII* can be delivered intercellularly through exosomes from glioma cells to nearby cells lacking this mutant form, which in turn leads to activation of transforming signaling pathways [34]. A further example of oncogene transfer was reported by Demory and colleagues, where exosomes extracted from a *KRAS* mutant cell line containing mutant KRAS protein resulted in internalization of the mutant isoform by wild-type CRC cells, and subsequent transformation [35].

There is emerging evidence that cancer-derived exosomes contribute to the recruitment and reprogramming of constituents associated with tumor environment, facilitating the so-called pre-metastatic niche. The pre-metastatic niche represents a specialized microenvironment that forms at the sites of future metastases and promotes the survival and outgrowth of disseminated cancer cells. This was reported in an in vivo pancreatic cancer model several years ago [36] and more recently Peinado and colleagues demonstrated that melanoma cell-derived exosomes are capable of recruiting bone-marrow-derived cells to initiate a pre-metastatic niche [37]. These and other data (reviewed in [38]) make a compelling case for the involvement of exosomes in the conditioning of the tumor microenvironment.

As regards immune system interactions, data suggest that exosomes have a broad role including modulating antigen presentation, immune activation, immune suppression, immune surveillance, and intercellular communication. It is acknowledged that during the neoplastic process, repression of adaptive immunity against cancer cells occurs. The role of exosomes can be divided into three categories: activity on effector T cells; immune regulatory cells; and NK cells. Apoptosis via Fas/FasL interaction represents one of the major pathways controlling T cell homeostasis through the selective elimination of over-reactive Fas-expressing T cells [39]. It has been shown that exosomes derived from many different cell lines have the ability to release pro-apoptotic exosomes, carrying not only FasL but also TRAIL on their surface [40–42]. This could also be shown with exosomes isolated from biological fluids, such as plasma and ascetic fluid [43, 44], ascribing to this mechanism a potential relevance in cancer patients.

Impact of cancer-derived exosomes on immune regulatory cells includes impaired dendritic cell differentiation [45] and promotion of MDSC differentiation from myeloid precursors [46]. Lastly, exosomes have been shown to inhibit the cytotoxicity of NK cells via NKG2D [47, 48].

Taken together, the data point to an important role for tumor-derived exosomes in promoting a pro-tumorigenic phenotype and facilitating immunosuppression.

Diagnostic Use

Any clinically useful diagnostic should have the following qualities: ease of accessibility for repeated or longitudinal sampling; carry information that is comprehensive; reflect the disease state in real time; and finally be amenable to high-throughput analysis. Arguably, exosomes meet all of these criteria. For these reasons they have become the focus of efforts to develop and bring to market liquid biopsy solutions that are either complementary to, or possibly even supplanting, tissue-based diagnostics.

As described above, exosomes are released from the cell surface by fusion of MVBs, resulting in vesicles that contain cytosolic components and expose the extracellular domain of some plasma membrane receptors at their surface. They are therefore a snapshot, or fingerprint, of the releasing cell and its status. Such a comprehensive and real-time insight into cellular function, in conjunction with their innate stability, clearly positions exosomes as crucial analytes in noninvasive diagnostics.

Exosomal Nucleic Acids as Biomarkers

Noninvasive Genotyping

The ability to assay nucleic acids from the circulation in several disease states is now well established. One of the earliest applications of cfDNA analysis has been in noninvasive prenatal testing (NIPT), typically in the identification of aneuploidy, and also in fetal mutation detection. Although not FDA approved, these approaches are commercially available and broadly accepted by the medical community [49].

An obvious application for the same technology is in oncology, as a means of genotyping a patient without the need for invasive biopsy. Until recently, identification of driver mutations for which approved targeted therapies are available required tissue-based analysis, obtained either at open biopsy or by percutaneous biopsy techniques. Neither approach is ideal or even suitable for the majority of common solid tumors: the majority of patients do not have readily biopsiable lesions, even assuming a patient's consent to an invasive procedure. For these reasons, the analysis of circulating tumor DNA (ctDNA) has in this area been gaining considerable ground.

The quantity of ctDNA that is available for analysis from a single blood draw (typically <25 mL whole blood) is variable, and dependent on the tumor of origin and the clinical stage of disease. Battachawa and colleagues [50] have demonstrated elegantly that even in the setting of stage IV disease, some tumor types yield very little circulating tumor DNA (ctDNA), often <20 copies/mL plasma, against a background of wild-type genes. The authors also demonstrate that abundance of ctDNA is tumor dependent, with gliomas less likely to shed nucleic acids into the general circulation, and colorectal and ovarian tumors considerably more so.

Exosomes have been shown to harbor these mutations on the RNA fraction contained intra-vesicularly [51]. In addition the biological source of exosomal RNA and cfDNA is entirely distinct: in contrast to cell-free DNA (cfDNA), which is released from apoptotic and necrotic bodies in a dying process of cells, exosomes are shed by living cells and arguably have greater relevance to ongoing cellular processes.

An example of a tumor type that is on the higher end of the range of cancers that shed cfDNA into the circulation is non-small-cell lung cancer (NSCLC), a disease for which a number of driver mutations are now well characterized, and for which corresponding targeted therapies are approved. Not surprisingly, a major effort has been under way to allow noninvasive genotyping in NSCLC, predominantly adenocarcinoma subtype, to obviate the need for invasive biopsies, yet reliably identify those harboring driver mutations. Several companies now offer this service in

CLIA-certified labs. Thus far, no liquid biopsy genotyping approach has been approved in oncology in the USA; however in September 2014, the EMA approved testing for *EGFR*-activating mutations (exons 19 and 21) using the Therascreen test on patient plasma [52]. This is the first such approval by a major regulatory body.

One class of mutations that has become important when considering targeted therapies in NSCLC, and beyond, is gene fusions. A well-established example would be *EML4-ALK* rearrangements in adenocarcinoma of the lung, first described by Soda and colleagues [53]. This fusion gene product, prevalent at 3–7% of NSCLC, almost exclusively adenocarcinoma, was subsequently shown to be a highly tractable target from a drug development point of view. The first approved ALK inhibitor, crizotinib, showed very high response rates as a single agent in ALK-positive NSCLC patients [54]; second- and third-generation inhibitors have since been developed. As with EGFR-activating mutation testing, the paradigm has thus far been tissue testing, either by FISH or IHC, the two FDA-approved assays [55]. EML4-ALK fusion gene product has however been shown to be detectable in exosomal RNA [56]. Indeed conceptually RNA analysis may be the best method of detection from a liquid biopsy point of view: searching for a slice variant or gene fusion on the DNA level requires considerable sequencing power, while exosomal RNA analysis can utilize simple qPCR. Performance characteristics have been presented for such a PCR-based exosomal RNA EML4-ALK plasma-based assay [57, 58]. An exosomal RNA plasma-based test is now commercially available [59].

One important consideration in noninvasive genotyping generally is maximization of sensitivity of detection. When compared to mutation detection on tumor tissue, the current gold standard, there is a moderate but very real false-negative rate, i.e., the positive concordance is less than 100%, and typically in the 60–70% range. The use of exosomes may be a way to address this "sensitivity gap." Recent experience in combining the capture and analysis of both exosomal RNA and cfDNA in order to maximize nucleic acid yield from biofluids, predominantly blood, has been presented [60]. The authors propose that by doing so, this maximizes sensitivity of detection of these so-called rare mutations, against a background of wild-type genes. Recently concordance data with tissue genotyping have been presented using this method for the detection of both EGFR-activating and *T790M* gatekeeper mutation in NSCLC, directly comparing an alternate liquid biopsy approach, using cfDNA [61].

RNA Signatures as Diagnostics

The ability to assay RNA from any biofluid is inherently hampered by its extreme lability: abundant and ubiquitous RNAses typically degrade any naked RNA almost instantaneously. miRNAs do exist in blood bound to and protected by Ago2 and other proteins or lipoproteins, but mRNA is not typically part of these complexes. Hence RNA expression profiling from a liquid biopsy has had to await robust and reproducible methods of isolation of exosomal RNA.

Recent work has shown the utility of this approach. McKiernan and colleagues recently published work on a three-gene RNA signature isolated from urinary exosomes [62]. In a large prospective trial, the signature was shown to predict the presence of high-grade (Gleason 6 or higher) prostate cancer in men over 50 presenting with a moderately elevated PSA presenting for a prostate biopsy. The urine sample does not require a DRE and is therefore completely noninvasive. The performance of the test, compared to the gold standard of prostatic biopsy, demonstrated an AUC of 0.71 and an NPV (the ability to accurately rule out the presence of high-grade cancer) in the 90% range. The test offers hope for avoiding unnecessary biopsies in a setting where PSA alone is very poorly discriminating. In a separate study, Eastham and colleagues have presented data showing that the three-gene signature, designated IntelliScore prostate, is significantly associated with stage and volume of disease at radical prostatectomy, and appears to discriminate disease progression post-surgery in a series of 359 patients [63]. The authors conclude however that further follow-up is required to confirm the observations.

Proteins as BMs

The protein content of exosomes from both patient samples and in vitro cell lines has been studied considerably. One area of interest has been in the early diagnosis of neurodegenerative disease. It has been reported that exosomal amyloid peptides accumulate in the brain plaques of Alzheimer's disease (AD) patients [64]. Furthermore, phospho-tau, an established biomarker for AD, is present at elevated levels in exosomes isolated from cerebrospinal fluid specimens of AD patients with mild symptoms [65]. These findings highlight the potential value of exosomes in the early diagnosis of AD, and may allow earlier therapeutic intervention in the disease process. Studies have also shown that α-synuclein, which plays a central role in Parkinson's disease, is released in exosomes in an in vitro PD model [66].

Recently, the cell surface proteoglycan, glypican-1, was identified as being specifically enriched on cancer exosomes. Monitoring glypican-1 on circulating exosomes demonstrated the ability to distinguish with encouraging specificity and sensitivity between healthy subjects and patients with benign pancreatic cancer from early- or late-stage pancreatic cancer patients [67]. Glypican-1 on circulating exosomes may prove to be an efficient noninvasive screening tool for pancreatic cancer, and holds out great hope for exosomes as cancer diagnostics.

Therapeutic Uses of Exosomes

Exosomes have many properties that recommend them as therapeutic vehicles: they are bioavailable, targetable to specific tissues, resistant to metabolic processes, and, perhaps most importantly, well tolerated given their role in normal physiology. A number of therapeutic strategies are viable, some of which have been tested in the clinic. Exosomes may be used to deliver an exogenous payload, such as a drug or toxin, and RNA, either modified or nascent, or manipulated to augment the immune response. These approaches are discussed below.

Regardless of the mode by which exosomes are utilized, a major challenge will be their robust and scalable production, as will be required to meet regulatory requirements.

A number of nanocarriers using various materials have been developed for drug delivery systems. Polyethylene glycol (PEG)-coated liposomes, which are frequently used as carriers for in vivo drug delivery, benefit from easy preparation techniques, acceptable toxicity profiles, and a lack of clearance by the reticuloendothelial system. Liposomes, however, do not generally lend themselves well to tissue targeting, and are associated with acute and occasionally severe hypersensitivity reactions.

An early indicator of the therapeutic potential of exosomes came from studies of cardiovascular ischemia, where it was observed that exosomes secreted by mesenchymal cells (MSCs) reduce reperfusion injury in the setting of acute myocardial infarction [68]. This has led to the exploration of MSCs as possible exosome "factories," which could be harvested and used therapeutically. Recently Pascucci has applied this approach to an in vivo pancreatic cancer model [69]. The authors found that MSCs can acquire strong antitumor activity after priming with paclitaxel through their capacity to uptake and then release the drug. This is the first demonstration that MSCs are able to package and deliver active drugs through their MVs. The same principle has been applied to chemotherapy-carrying exosomes in a breast cancer model [70]. To reduce immunogenicity and toxicity, mouse immature dendritic cells (imDCs) were used for exosome production. Notably, tumor targeting was facilitated by engineering the imDCs to express a well-characterized exosomal membrane protein (Lamp2b) fused to αv integrin-specific iRGD peptide. The authors showed that intravenously injected targeted exosomes delivered doxorubicin specifically to tumor tissues, leading to inhibition of tumor growth without overt toxicity.

A related though inverse observation has been made by Federici and colleagues, who show that a possible mechanism of platinum drug resistance is via drug extrusion within exosomes [71].

The polyphenol, curcumin, has been under investigation for some time, and has been reported to have anti-inflammatory and antitumor activities [72, 73]. Interestingly, curcumin also reduces the inhibitory effects of exosomes on NK cytotoxicity [74]. The poor solubility of curcumin has generally limited its usefulness, although its bioavailability can be enhanced by its encapsulation in liposomes [75]. However, the delivery of curcumin by exosomes was found to be much more effective than liposomal delivery by preventing septic shock [76].

Yang and colleagues recently tested the hypothesis that brain endothelial cell-derived exosomes can deliver anticancer drug across the BBB for the treatment of brain cancer in a zebrafish (*Danio rerio*) model [77]. The authors suggest that brain endothelial cell-derived exosomes could be potentially used as a carrier for brain delivery of anticancer drug for the treatment of brain cancer, thereby addressing the BBB issue.

Due to their viral-like transfection efficiency and inherent biological function, compelling evidence indicates that exosomes can be used as novel delivery platforms for RNA, including miRNA. Alvarez-Elviti and colleagues have reported on the use of exosomes to transport short interfering (si)RNA to the brain in mice [78]. To reduce immunogenicity, the authors used self-derived dendritic cells for exosome production. The therapeutic potential of exosome-mediated siRNA delivery was demonstrated by the strong mRNA (60%) and protein (62%) knockdown of BACE1, a therapeutic target in Alzheimer's disease, in wild-type mice. In order to test whether marrow stromal cell (MSC) exosomes could be used as a vehicle for delivery of antitumor miRNAs, Katakowski and colleagues transfected MSCs with a miR-146b expression plasmid, and harvested exosomes released by the MSCs [79]. Intra-tumor injection of exosomes derived from miR-146-expressing MSCs significantly reduced glioma xenograft growth in a rat model of primary brain tumor.

Lastly, exosomes may be utilized as a way of presenting vesicle-bound antigens, representing a new cancer vaccine strategy [80]. In addition, Gehrmann and coworkers explored induction of adaptive antitumor immunity by co-delivery of antigen with α-galactosylceramide on exosomes [81]. Their findings show that exosomes loaded with protein antigen and αGC will activate adaptive immunity in the absence of triggering iNKT-cell anergy, supporting their application in the design of a broad variety of cancer immunotherapy trials.

In summary, as they are nonviable, the risk profile of exosomes is thought to be less than that of cellular therapies. Exosomes can be manufactured at scale in culture, and exosomes can be engineered to incorporate therapeutic miRNAs, siRNAs, or chemotherapeutic molecules. At the current time, System Biosciences, Inc. offers a commercially available kit, XPack™, which allows for cell-mediated generation of ready-to-use exosomes packed with any protein of choice, for research use [82]. These exosomes can then be used to efficiently deliver proteins to target cells to alter or supplement biological pathways or be used to study exosome trafficking in vivo.

A potential advance on targeting of exosomes and their payloads was recently reported by Hung et al. using engineered glycosylation thereby stabilizing the surface proteins [83].

Clinical Trials of Exosome-Based Therapy

At the time of writing, a search on Clinicaltrials.gov using the term "exosome" returned 28 studies, of which 6 were interventional trials. One of the most extensively published approaches involves the use of dexosomes, exosomes derived from dendritic cells. Early work using this procedure was by Morse and coworkers [84]. They performed this study to test the safety, feasibility, and efficacy of autologous dendritic cell (DC)-derived exosomes (DEX) loaded with the MAGE tumor antigens in patients with NSCLC. They conclude that production of the DEX vaccine was feasible and DEX therapy was well tolerated in patients with advanced NSCLC. Some patients experienced long-term stability of disease and activation of immune effectors. A similar approach has been pursued in melanoma [85].

Conclusions

The number of peer-reviewed publications focused on exosomes has increased exponentially over the last 15 years, and our understanding of exosome biology has increased correspondingly. Having seen the launch of the first exosome-based DLT diagnostic in 2016 for the detection of *EML4-ALK* mutations in NSCLC, we are now poised to witness an expansion of diagnostic applications within oncology, and beyond. Further, the therapeutic possibilities of exosomes are being aggressively pursued. It is not unlikely that over the next few years, exosomes will become a required analyte for liquid biopsy approaches, and a standard delivery system for small molecules and nucleic acids.

References

1. Pan B-T, Johnstone RM (1983) Fate of the transferrin receptor during maturation of sheep reticulocytes in vitro: selective externalization of the receptor. Cell 33(3):967–977
2. Pan B-T, Teng K, Wu C, Adam A, Johnstone RM (1985) Electron microscopic evidence for externalization of the transferrin receptor in vesicular form in sheep reticulocytes. J Cell Biol 101(3):942–948
3. Friend C, Marovitz W, Henie G, Henie W, Tsuei D, Hirschhorn K, Holland JG, Cuttner J (1978) Observations on cell lines derived from a patient with hodgkin's disease. Cancer Res 38:2581–2591
4. Van Blitterswijk WJ, Emmelot P, Hilkmann HA, Hilgers J, Feltkamp CA (1979) Rigid plasma-membrane-derived vesicles, enriched in tumour-associated surface antigens (MLR), occurring in the ascites fluid of a murine leukaemia (GRSL). Int J Cancer 23:62–70
5. Zhang J, Li S, Li L, Li M, Guo C, Yao J, Mi S (2015) Exosome and exosomal MicroRNA: trafficking, sorting, and function. Genomics Proteomics Bioinformatics 13(1):17–24
6. Qiagen Website. http://sabiosciences.com/manuals/seminars/Exosomes_exoEasy_exoR-Neasy.pdf
7. Miyanishi M, Tada K, Koike M, Uchiyama Y, Kitamura T, Nagata S (2007) Identification of Tim4 as a phosphatidylserine receptor. Nature 450(7168):435–439
8. Deng ZB, Zhuang X, Ju S, Xiang X, Mu J, Liu Y, Jiang H, Zhang L, Mobley J, McClain C, Feng W, Grizzle W, Yan J, Miller D, Kronenberg M, Zhang HG (2013) Exosome-like nanoparticles from intestinal mucosal cells carry prostaglandin E2 and suppress activation of liver NKT cells. J Immunol 190(7):3579–3589
9. Valadi H, Ekstrom K, Bossios A, Sjostrand M, Lee JJ, Lotvall JO (2007) Exosome-mediated transfer of mRNAs and microRNAs is a novel mechanism of genetic exchange between cells. Nat Cell Biol 9(6):654–659
10. Skog J, Würdinger T, Van Rijn S et al (2008) Glioblastoma microvesicles transport RNA and proteins that promote tumour growth and provide diagnostic biomarkers. Nat Cell Biol 10(12):1470–1476

11. Hunter MP, Ismail N, Zhang X, Aguda BD, Lee EJ, Yu L, Xiao T, Schafer J, Lee ML, Schmittgen TD, Nana-Sinkam SP, Jarjoura D, Marsh CB (2008) Detection of microRNA expression in human peripheral blood microvesicles. PLoS One 3(11):e3694
12. Rabinowits G, Gerçel-Taylor C, Day JM, Taylor DD, Kloecker GH (2009) Clin Exosomal microRNA: a diagnostic marker for lung cancer. Lung Cancer 10(1):42–46
13. Michael A, Bajracharya SD, Yuen PS, Zhou H, Star RA et al (2010) Exosomes from human saliva as a source of microRNA biomarkers. Oral Dis 16:34–38
14. Nilsson J, Skog J, Nordstrand A et al (2009) Prostate cancer-derived urine exosomes: a novel approach to biomarkers for prostate cancer. Br J Cancer 100(10):1603–1607
15. van der Pol E, Böing AN, Harrison P, Sturk A, Nieuwland R (2012) Classification, functions, and clinical relevance of extracellular vesicles. Pharmacol Rev 64(3):676–705
16. http://exocarta.org/
17. Chen K, Rajewsky N (2007) The evolution of gene regulation by transcription factors and microRNAs. Nat Rev Genet 8:93–103
18. Esquela-Kerscher A, Slack FJ (2006) Oncomirs—microRNAs with a role in cancer. Nat Rev Cancer 6:259–269
19. Calin GA, Croce CM (2006) MicroRNA signatures in human cancers. Nat Rev Cancer 6:857–866
20. Petrocca F, Lieberman J (2009) Micromanipulating cancer: microRNA-based therapeutics? RNA Biol 6:335–340
21. Tong AW, Nemunaitis J (2008) Modulation of miRNA activity in human cancer: a new paradigm for cancer gene therapy? Cancer Gene Ther 15:341–355
22. Zomer A, Vendrig T, Hopmans ES, Van Eijndhoven M, Middeldorp JM, Pegtel DM (2010) Exosomes: fit to deliver small RNA. Commun Integr Biol 3:447–450
23. Hong BS, Cho JH, Kim H, Choi EJ, Rho S, Kim J, Kim JH, Choi DS, Kim YK, Hwang D, Gho YS (2009) Colorectal cancer cell-derived microvesicles are enriched in cell cycle-related mRNAs that promote proliferation of endothelial cells. BMC Genomics 10:556
24. Skog J, Wurdinger T, Van Rijn S, Meijer DH, Gainche L, Sena-Esteves M, Curry WT Jr, Carter BS, Krichevsky AM, Breakefield XO (2008) Glioblastoma microvesicles transport RNA and proteins that promote tumour growth and provide diagnostic biomarkers. Nat Cell Biol 10:1470–1476
25. Mathivanan S, Ji H, Simpson RJ (2010) Exosomes: extracellular organelles important in intercellular communication. J Proteome 73:1907–1920
26. Simpson RJ, Lim JW, Moritz RL, Mathivanan S (2009) Exosomes: proteomic insights and diagnostic potential. Expert Rev Proteomics 6:267–283
27. Adamczyk KA, Klein-Scory S, Tehrani MM, Warnken U, Schmiegel W, Schnolzer M, Schwarte-Waldhoff I (2011) Characterization of soluble and exosomal forms of the EGFR released from pancreatic cancer cells. Life Sci 89:304–316
28. Pisitkun T, Shen RF, Knepper MA (2004) Identification and proteomic profiling of exosomes in human urine. Proc Natl Acad Sci U S A 101(36):13368–13373
29. Gonzales PA, Pisitkun T, Hoffert JD, Tchapyjnikov D, Star RA, Kleta R, Wang NS, Knepper MA (2009) Large-scale proteomics and phosphoproteomics of urinary exosomes. J Am Soc Nephrol 20(2):363–379
30. https://hpcwebapps.cit.nih.gov/ESBL/Database/Exosome/
31. Hannafon BN, Ding WQ (2013) Intercellular communication by exosome-derived microRNAs in cancer. Int J Mol Sci 14(7):14240–14269
32. Record M, Carayon K, Poirot M, Silvente-Poirot S (2014) Exosomes as new vesicular lipid transporters involved in cell-cell communication and various pathophysiologies. Biochim Biophys Acta 1841(1):108–120
33. Zakharova L, Svetlova M, Fomina AF (2007) T cell exosomes induce cholesterol accumulation in human monocytes via phosphatidylserine receptor. J Cell Physiol 212(1):174–181
34. Al-Nedawi K, Meehan B, Micallef J, Lhotak V, May L, Guha A, Rak J (2008) Intercellular transfer of the oncogenic receptor EGFRvIII by microvesicles derived from tumour cells. Nat Cell Biol 10(5):619–624

35. Demory Beckler M, Higginbotham JN, Franklin JL, Ham AJ, Halvey PJ, Imasuen IE, Whitwell C, Li M, Liebler DC, Coffey RJ (2012) Proteomic analysis of exosomes from mutant KRAS colon cancer cells identifies intercellular transfer of mutant KRAS. Mol Cell Proteomics 12(2):343–355. doi:10.1074/mcp.M112.022806

36. Jung T, Castellana D, Klingbeil P, Cuesta Hernandez I, Colonna M, Orlicky DJ, Roffler SR, Brodt P, Zoller M (2009) CD44v6 dependence of premetastatic niche preparation by exosomes. Neoplasia 11(10):1093–1105

37. Peinado H, Aleckovic M, Lavotshkin S, Matei I, Costa-Silva B, Moreno-Bueno G, Hergueta-Redondo M, Williams C, Garcia-Santos G, Ghajar C, Nitadori-Hoshino A, Hoffman C (2012) Melanoma exosomes educate bone marrow progenitor cells toward a pro-metastatic phenotype through MET. Nat Med 18(6):883–891

38. Alderton GK (2012 Jul) Metastasis. Exosomes drive premetastatic niche formation. Nat Rev Cancer 12(7):447

39. Osborne BA (1996) Apoptosis and the maintenance of homoeostasis in the immune system. Curr Opin Immunol 8:245–254

40. Bergmann C, Strauss L, Wieckowski E, Czystowska M, Albers A, Wang Y et al (2009) Tumor-derived microvesicles in sera of patients with head and neck cancer and their role in tumor progression. Head Neck 31:371–380

41. Martinez-Lorenzo MJ, Anel A, Alava MA, Pineiro A, Naval J, Lasierra P et al (2004) The human melanoma cell line MelJuSo secretes bioactive FasL and APO2L/TRAIL on the surface of microvesicles. Possible contribution to tumor counterattack. Exp Cell Res 295:315–329

42. Qu JL, Qu XJ, Qu JL, Qu XJ, Zhao MF, Teng YE et al (2009) The role of cbl family of ubiquitin ligases in gastric cancer exosome-induced apoptosis of Jurkat T cells. Acta Oncol 48:1173–1180

43. Wieckowski EU, Visus C, Szajnik M, Szczepanski MJ, Storkus WJ, Whiteside TL (2009) Tumor-derived microvesicles promote regulatory T cell expansion and induce apoptosis in tumor-reactive activated CD8+ T lymphocytes. J Immunol 183:3720–3730

44. Peng P, Yan Y, Keng S (2011) Exosomes in the ascites of ovarian cancer patients: origin and effects on anti-tumor immunity. Oncol Rep 25:749–762

45. Gabrilovich DI, Nagaraj S (2009) Myeloid-derived suppressor cells as regulators of the immune system. Nat Rev Immunol 9:162–174

46. Valenti R, Huber V, Filipazzi P, Pilla L, Sovena G, Villa A et al (2006) Human tumorreleased microvesicles promote the differentiation of myeloid cells with transforming growth factor-beta-mediated suppressive activity on T lymphocytes. Cancer Res 66:9290–9298

47. Clayton A, Tabi Z (2005) Exosomes and the MICA-NKG2D system in cancer. Blood Cells Mol Dis 34:206–213

48. Clayton A, Mitchell JP, Court J, Linnane S, Mason MD, Tabi Z (2008) Human tumor-derived exosomes down-modulate NKG2D expression. J Immunol 180:7249–7258

49. https://www.sequenom.com/tests/reproductive-health

50. Bettegowda C, Sausen M, Leary RJ, Kinde I, Wang Y, Agrawal N et al (2014) Detection of circulating tumor DNA in early- and late-stage human malignancies. Sci Transl Med 6(224):224

51. Chen WW, Balaj L, Liau LM, Samuels ML, Kotsopoulos SK, Maguire CA, Loguidice L, Soto H, Garrett M, Zhu LD, Sivaraman S, Chen C, Wong ET, Carter BS, Hochberg FH, Breakefield XO, Skog J (2013) BEAMing and droplet digital PCR analysis of mutant IDH1 mRNA in glioma patient serum and cerebrospinal fluid extracellular vesicles. Mol Ther Nucleic Acids 2:e109

52. Qiagen Press Release (2015)

53. Soda M, Choi YL, Enomoto M et al (2007) Identification of the transforming EML4-ALK fusion gene in non-small-cell lung cancer. Nature 448:561–566

54. Kwak EL, Bang YJ, Camidge DR et al (2010) Anaplastic lymphoma kinase inhibition in non-small-cell lung cancer. N Engl J Med 363:1693–1703

55. www.fda.gov

56. Brinkmann K, Enderle D, Koestler T, Bentink S, Emenegger J, Spiel A, Mueller R, O'Neill V, Skog J, Noerholm M (2006) Plasma-based diagnostics for detection of EML4-ALK fusion transcripts in NSCLC patients [abstract]. In: Proceedings of the annual meeting of the American Association for Cancer Research, Washington, DC, AACR, 1–5 Apr 2006, Abstract nr 545

57. O'Neill, V, Brinkmann K, Skog J (2016) Exosomal RNA based liquid biopsy detection of EML4-ALK in plasma from NSCLC patients. Proceedings from the annual meeting of the NCCN. Ft Lauderdale, FL, 2016. Abstract No: 42

58. Brinkmann K, Carbone DP, Enderle D, Koestler T, Bentink S, Emenegger J, Spiel A, Mueller R, O'Neill V, Skog J, Noerholm M (2015) Exosomal RNA based liquid biopsy detection of EML4-ALK in plasma from NSCLC patients (ID 2591). Proceedings from the International Association IALSC, Denver, Colorado

59. www.exosomedx.com

60. Enderle D, Koestler T, Spiel A, Brinkmann K, Bentink S, Skog J, Noerholm M (2014) Development of a single-step isolation platform to analyze exosomal RNA and cell-free DNA in plasma from cancer patients. EORTC-NCI-AACR 2014. Abstract No 313

61. A.K. Krug, C. Karlovich, T. Koestler, S. Bentink, K. Brinkmann, A. Spiel, J. Emenegger, M. Noerholm, V. O'Neill, L.V. Sequist, JC. Soria, J.W. Goldman, D. Ross Camidge, H.A. Wakelee, S.M. Gadgeel, E. Mann, S. Matheny, L. Rolfe, M. Raponi, D. Enderle, J. Skog (2015) Plasma EGFR mutation detection using a combined exosomal RNA and circulating tumor DNA approach in patients with acquired resistance to first-generation EGFR-TKIs. 26th AACR-NCI-EORTC International conference on molecular targets and cancer therapeutics in Boston, Mass

62. McKiernan J, Donovan MJ, O'Neill V, et al. A novel urine exosome gene expression assay to predict high-grade prostate cancer at initial biopsy. JAMA Oncol 2:882-889 Published online March 2016.

63. Eastham J, Donovan D, Patel V, O'Neill V, Bentink S, Skog J, James McKiernan JM (2016) Preliminary assessment of a validated urine exosome assay (ExDx Prostate (IntelliScore) for predicting biochemical recurrence post-prostatectomy. American Urology Association Meeting, San Diego, CA, 2016. Plenary Abstract

64. Rajendran L, Honsho M, Zahn TR et al (2006) Alzheimer's disease B-amyloid peptides are released in association with exosomes. Proc Natl Acad Sci U S A 103(30):11172–11177

65. Saman S, Kim W, Raya M et al (2012) Exosome-associated tau is secreted in tauopathy models and is selectively phosphorylated in cerebrospinal fluid in early Alzheimer disease. J Biol Chem 287(6):3842–3849

66. Alvarez-Erviti L, Seow Y, Schapira AH et al (2011) Lysosomal dysfunction increases exosome-mediated alpha-synuclein release and transmission. Neurobiol Dis 42(3):360–367

67. Melo SA, Luecke LB, Kahlert C, Fernandez AF, Gammon ST, Kaye J, LeBleu VS, Mittendorf EA, Weitz J, Rahbari N et al (2015) Glypican-1 identifies cancer exosomes and detects early pancreatic cancer. Nature 523:177–182

68. Lai RC, Arslan F, Lee MM et al (2010) Exosome secreted by MSC reduces myocardial ischemia/reperfusion injury. Stem Cell Res 4:214–222

69. Pascucci L, Coccè V, Bonomi A, Ami D, Ceccarelli P, Ciusani E, Viganò L, Locatelli A, Sisto F, Doglia SM et al (2014) Paclitaxel is incorporated by mesenchymal stromal cells and released in exosomes that inhibit in vitro tumor growth: a new approach for drug delivery. J Control Release 192:262–270

70. Tian Y, Li S, Song J, Ji T, Zhu M, Anderson GJ, Wei J, Nie G (2014) A doxorubicin delivery platform using engineered natural membrane vesicle exosomes for targeted tumor therapy. Biomaterials 35:2383–2390

71. Federici C, Petrucci F, Caimi S, Cesolini A, Logozzi M, Borghi M, D'Ilio S, Lugini L, Violante N, Azzarito T et al (2014) Exosome release and low pH belong to a framework of resistance of human melanoma cells to cisplatin. PLoS One 9:e88193

72. Narayan S (2004) Curcumin, a multi-functional chemopreventive agent, blocks growth of colon cancer cells by targeting β-catenin-mediated transactivation and cell-cell adhesion pathways. J Mol Histol 35:301–307

73. Jaiswal AS, Marlow BP, Gupta N, Narayan S (2002) β-Catenin-mediated transactivation and cell-cell adhesion pathways are important in curcumin (diferuylmethan)-induced growth arrest and apoptosis in colono cancer cells. Oncogene 21:8414–8427

74. Zhang HG, Kim H, Liu C, Yu S, Wang J, Grizzle WE et al (1773) Curcumin reverses breast tumor exosomes mediated immune suppression of NK cell tumor cytotoxicity. Biochim Biophys Acta 2007:1116–1123

75. Narayanan NK, Nargi D, Randolph C, Narayanan BA (2009) Liposome encapsulation of curcumin and resveratrol in combination reduces prostate cancer incidence in PTEN knockout mice. Int J Cancer 125:1–8

76. Sun D, Zhuang X, Xiang X, Liu Y, Zhang S, Liu C et al (2010) A novel nanoparticle drug delivery system. The anti-inflammatory activity of curcumin is enhanced when encapsulated in exosomes. Mol Ther 18:1606–1614

77. Yang T, Martin P, Fogarty B, Brown A, Schurman K, Phipps R, Yin VP, Lockman P, Bai S (2015) Exosome delivered anticancer drugs across the blood-brain barrier for brain cancer therapy in *Danio rerio*. Pharm Res 32:2003–2014

78. Alvarez-Erviti L, Seow Y, Yin H, Betts C, Lakhal S, Wood MJ (2011) Delivery of siRNA to the mouse brain by systemic injection of targeted exosomes. Nat Biotechnol 29:341–345

79. Katakowski M, Buller B, Zheng X, Lu Y, Rogers T, Osobamiro O, Shu W, Jiang F, Chopp M (2013) Exosomes from marrow stromal cells expressing miR-146b inhibit glioma growth. Cancer Lett 335:201–204

80. Lee EY, Park KS, Yoon YJ, Lee J, Moon HG, Jang SC, Choi KH, Kim YK, Gho YS (2012) Therapeutic effects of autologous tumor-derived nanovesicles on melanoma growth and metastasis. PLoS One 7:e33330

81. Gehrmann U, Hiltbrunner S, Georgoudaki AM, Karlsson MC, Naslund TI, Gabrielsson S (2013) Synergistic induction of adaptive antitumor immunity by co-delivery of antigen with alpha-galactosylceramide on exosomes. Cancer Res 73:3865–3876

82. Systems biosciences website. https://www.systembio.com/xpack-exosomes/overview

83. Hung ME, Leonard JN (2015) Stabilization of exosome-targeting peptides via engineered glycosylation. J Biol Chem 290:8166–8172

84. Morse MA, Garst J, Osada T, Khan S, Hobeika A, Clay TM, Valente N, Shreeniwas R, Sutton MA, Delcayre A, Hsu DH, Le Pecq JB, Lyerly HK (2005 Feb 21) A phase I study of dexosome immunotherapy in patients with advanced non-small cell lung cancer. J Transl Med 3(1):9

85. www.clinicaltrials.gov. NCT00042497

Index

A

AdnaTest® (Qiagen, Germany), 44, 45
Adriamycin, 25
Aldehyde dehydrogenase (ALDH), 125
Aldehyde dehydrogenase 1 (ALDH1), 70
Alzheimer's disease (AD), 148
Amoeboid-cell migration, 68
Amplification refractory mutation system
    (ARMS), 109
Androgen receptor (AR), 6, 113
Angiogenic phenotype, 25
Anoikis, 21, 22
Anticancer agents, 2

B

β-actin, 45
Beads, emulsions, amplifications, magnetics
    (BEAMing), 108–110, 112
Bioanalyzer electrophoresis approach, 45
Biomarker analysis in cancer, 94
Biomarkers
    exosomal nucleic acids as
        noninvasive genotyping, 146, 147
    in peripheral blood, 4
        CTCs, 5, 6
        ctDNA, 7, 8
        exosomes, 8
Blood-based biopsy (BBB), 82, 84, 95–97
Blood-derived biopsy
    advantages and challenges, 120
BM biopsy, 19
Bone marrow
    DTCs, 24
BRAF V600 mutation, 130

C

Cancer stem cells (CSCs), 2, 18, 25
    complete and partial EMT, 70
    metastasis, 70
Cancer treatment, future, 94, 95
Cancer-associated fibroblasts (CAFs), 84,
    89, 90
Cancer-associated macrophage-like (CAMLs)
    cells, 85, 86, 91
Cancer-associated macrophage-like cell, 87
Cancer-associated neutrophils (CANs),
    89, 90
Carcinoembryonic antigen (CEA), 96
Carcinoma-associated fibroblasts (CAFs), 69
Cargo sorting, 144
CellCollector™, 45
Cell-free circulating DNA (ccfDNA), 127
Cell-free DNA (cfDNA), 105, 107, 146
    sources of, 107, 108
    technologies to measure, 108, 109
CellSearch platform, 121–124
CellSearch test, 124
CellSearch® CEC assay, 88
CellSearch® system, 5, 44, 48, 53–55, 75
CellSieve™ microfilters, 85, 95, 96
CellSieve™ microfiltration, 87
Centrifugation, 47
Cerebral spinal fluid (CSF), 107, 111
Chemotherapy, 68

Breast cancer (BrCa), 15, 41, 48, 68
    metastatic (*see* Metastatic BrCa)
Breast cancer metastasis suppressor 1
    (*BRMS1*), 53

© Springer International Publishing AG 2017
M. Cristofanilli (ed.), *Liquid Biopsies in Solid Tumors*, Cancer Drug Discovery
and Development, DOI 10.1007/978-3-319-50956-3

157

Circulating cancer-associated macrophage-like
        (CAMLs), 87, 88
Circulating cancer-associated vascular
        endothelial cells (CAVEs), 85, 86,
        88, 89, 91
Circulating cell-free DNA (cfDNA), 7, 93, 120
Circulating endothelial cells (CECs), 88
Circulating epithelial cells (CECs), 125
Circulating Free Tumor DNA (ctDNA),
        111–114
    clinical applications
        early-stage cancer, 112, 113
        metastatic cancer, 113, 114
        prevention and screening, 111
    concordance studies, 109–111
Circulating stromal cells (CStCs), 82,
        84–87, 91
    cancer mass with, 82
    presence and prevalence of CTCs and,
        90, 92
Circulating tumor cells (CTCs)
    cancer mass with, 82
    characterisation, 27, 30
    clinical applications, 26, 27
    clinical studies, 28–29
    enrichment, isolation and detection
        systems, 43, 57
        centrifugation, 47
        DEP, 47
        functional assays, 48
        imaging systems, 47, 48
        in vivo positive, 45
        microfluidic based positive, 45
        by negative selection, 46
        positive immunomagnetic selection,
            44, 45
        size- and/or deformability-based,
            46, 47
    enumeration, 121
    evidence, 120
    experimental approaches, 121
    form and function, boundaries, 125–127
    functional, 121, 122
    impact, 123–125
    interventional studies, 30, 31
    metastasis, 68, 69, 71
        complete and partial EMT, 72, 73
        regulating EMT and CSC properties,
            73, 74
        as traveling diagnostic and target,
            74, 75
    metastatic BrCa
        clinical significance of CTC
            enumeration, 48–50
        molecular characterization, 51–54

metastatic cascade, 19
    circulation and extravasation, 21–24
    formation of metastasis, 24–26
    local invasion and intravasation,
        19–21
metastatic site, 121
models of metastatic progression, 16
    linear and parallel progression, 16–18
    tumour Self-Seeding, 18, 19
molecular, 121–123
and nucleic acids, 120
presence and prevalence of CStCs and,
    90, 92
prevalence, 91
primary tumour, 30
prognostic factors, 26, 27
prognostic value, 121
QC, 55, 57
utility, 121
Circulating tumor DNA (ctDNA), 7, 93, 127,
        128, 146
    boundaries by detection tools,
        128–130
Circulating tumor materials (CTMat), 4
Circulating tumor microemboli (CTM), 6
Clinical applications
    early-stage cancer, 112, 113
    metastatic cancer, 113, 114
    prevention and screening, 111
Clonal evolution theory, 2
Clonal heterogeneity, 3
Clustered circulating tumour cells,
        22, 23
c-Myc, 74
Collective-cell migration, 69
CTC enumeration, 44
CTC-Chip, 45
CTC-iChip, 45
Curcumin, 149
Cystatin E/M, 53
CytoTrack™ system, 47

D
Density-based gradient centrifugation, 47
DEPArray™ (Menarini Diagnostics)
        platform, 47
DEPArray™ systems, 54
Dielectrophoresis (DEP), 47
Disseminated tumour cells (DTCs), 4, 15, 24
Distant disease-free survival (DDFS), 27
Dormancy, 16, 24–25
Driver mutations, 2
Droplet digital PCR (ddPCR), 108
Ductal carcinoma in situ (DCIS), 17

E
E-cadherin (CDH1), 74
EGFR, 22
Enrichment techniques, 5
EpCAM-based method, 20, 21
Epidermal growth factor (EGF), 20
Epithelial cell adhesion molecule (EpCAM),
    42, 75, 86, 122, 124
EPIthelial immunoSPOT (EPISPOT), 48
Epithelial-mesenchymal transition (EMT), 16,
    19–21, 29, 68, 122
  complete and partial, CSC, 70
  metastasis, 68, 69
ExoCarta, 142, 143
Exosomal shuttle RNA (esRNA), 141
Exosomes
  biogenesis, 141
  classes of molecules, 141
  clinical trials, 150–151
  diagnostic use, 145
  discovery, 140
  exosomal nucleic acids as biomarkers
      noninvasive genotyping, 146, 147
  function, 144
  genesis, 140, 141
  lipids, 144
  miRNAs, 142, 143
  mRNA, 143
  proteins, 143
  proteins as BMs, 148
  RNA signatures as diagnostics, 147, 148
  structure and content, 141, 142
  therapeutic uses, 148–150
Extracellular matrix (ECM), 20, 68
Extracellular vesicles (EVs), 139

F
FASTCell™, 47
Ficoll-Paque®, 47
Flow cytometry, 85
Flow cytometry analysis, 87
Fluorescence-activated cytometers, 121
Functional assays, 48
  EPISPOT, 48
  leukapheresis, 48
  patient-derived xenografts, 48
Functionally structured medical nanowire
    (FSMW), 45

G
Geometrically enhanced differential
    immunocapture (GEDI), 45
Gold standard technologies, 55

H
Halstedian model, 16
HB (herringbone)-chip, 45
Heat-shock proteins (HSP70), 140
Hepatocyte growth factor (HGF) signalling
    pathways, 20
HER2 status discordance, 30
HER2-negative primary tumors, 49
HER2-positive CTCs, 49
Heterogeneity, 18
Hodgkin's disease, 140
Human epidermal growth factor receptor 2
    (HER2) gene, 18

I
Immature dendritic cells (imDCs), 149
Immune checkpoint therapies, 94, 95
Immunochemistry techniques, 5
Immunodeficient mice model, 22
In vivo positive enrichment technologies, 45
Individualized treatment, 57
Innovative Medicines Initiative (IMI), 57
Intercellular communication, 139
Isolated cell types, 86
Isolation by size of epithelial tumor cells
    (ISET), 46

K
KRAS protein, 144

L
Leukapheresis, 48
Leukemias, 106
Liposarcoma, 25
Liquid biopsies, 4, 8, 31, 42, 84, 93, 94, 96,
    97, 106, 109, 110, 113–115, 127,
    130, 145, 147, 151
Logistical sampling, 55
Loss of heterozygosity (LOH), 53
Luminex® analyzer, 52
Lymphoprep™, 47

M
MagSweeper, 45, 55
Mammospheres, 26
Marrow stromal cell (MSC), 150
Matrix metalloproteinases (MMPs), 68
Mesenchymal cells (MSCs), 149
Mesenchymal to epithelial transition
    (MET), 69
Metalloproteinases (MMP), 20

Metastasis, 41
Metastasis-initiating cells (MICs), 71
Metastatic BrCa, 51–54
    clinical significance of CTC enumeration,
        48–50
    molecular characterization of CTCs
        DNA methylation studies, 53, 54
        gene expression, 51, 52
        mutation detection studies, 53
    single-cell analysis, 54–56
Metastatic cancer, clinical applications,
    113, 114
Metastatic disease, 68
Microenvironment engineers, 20
Microfiltration systems, 46, 47
    ISET, 46
Microinvasive disease, 17
MicroRNAs (miRNAs), 142, 143
Microvesicles (MVs), 140
Minimal residual disease, 7
Molecular abnormalities in circulation, 93
Monocytes (MCs), 20
Multivesicular body (MVB), 140
Murine immortalised cells, 26
Murine model, 19
Mutated DNA, 93
Mutator hypothesis, 2

N
Negative selection technologies, 46
Next-generation sequencing (NGS), 8,
    108, 120
Noninvasive genotyping, 146, 147
Noninvasive prenatal testing (NIPT), 146
Non-small-cell lung cancer (NSCLC), 5, 146
Nucleic acid-based techniques, 5

O
OncoQuick®, 47
Osteosarcoma murine model, 19
Overdiagnosis, 111

P
Paracrine effect, 19
Parallel progression models, 18
Parkinson's disease, 106, 148
Parsortix® (Angle), 46
Patient-derived xenografts, 48
Peritoneovenous shunts, 21–22
Personalized medicine, 2
Phenotypical flexibility, 23

Phosphatidylinositol, 144
Phosphatidylserine, 141, 144
Photoacoustic flow cytometry (PAFC), 47
Plakoglobin, 23
Plasma tumor DNA (ptDNA), 107, 108, 110,
    112–114
    markers of prognosis, 113
    metastatic tissue, 110
    prognostic value, 113
    technologies to measure, 108, 109
    with tumor biopsy sequencing, 115
Plastic CSC model, 3
Podsypanina, 18
Polyethylene glycol (PEG)-coated
    liposomes, 149
Polyphenol, 149
Prospective randomized open blinded
    end-point (PROBE), 92
Prostate-specific antigen (PSA), 96, 111
Prostate-specific membrane antigen (PSMA), 88
Protein plakoglobin, 23

Q
Quality control (QC) in CTC analysis, 55, 57
Quenching, underivatizing, amine stripping,
    and restaining (QUAS-R), 92

R
Radiotherapy, 68
Red blood cell (RBC) lysis, 85
Reverse transcriptase polymerase chain
    reaction (RT-PCR), 30
Rho GTPases, 68
RosetteSep™ CTC Enrichment Cocktail, 47

S
ScreenCell® filters, 46
Self-seeding, 71
Sensitivity gap, 147
Single circulating tumour cells, 21, 22
Single CTC, 17
Single-cell analysis, 54–56
Skin cancers, 41
Solid tumors, 2
    stromal cells, 82–84
Southwest Oncology Group (SWOG), 49
SRY (sex-determining region Y)-box 17
    (SOX17), 54
Stemness, 16, 24–26
Stromal cells
    solid tumors, 82–84

T

T oncogene, 18
Tagged amplicon sequencing (TAm-Seq), 110
Targeted therapies, 94, 95
Tissue factors (TF), 69
Transforming growth factor beta (TGFbeta), 20
Trastuzumab, 31
Triple-negative breast cancer (TNBC), 25
Tumor biomarkers, 94, 130
Tumor dissemination, 69
Tumor endothelial cells (TECs), 84, 88, 89
Tumor heterogeneity, 2
    clonal evolution theory, 2
    CSC model, 2
    models, 3
    molecular resistance, 7
    mutator hypothesis, 2
    plastic CSC model, 3

Tumor-associated cells, 126
Tumor-associated macrophages
        (TAMs), 84
    circulating CAMLs, 87, 88
Tumor-initiating cells (TICs), 84,
        122, 125
Tumors
    diagnosis, 8
Tumour self-seeding, 18, 19
Tumour-initiating cell, 25

W

White blood cells (WBC), 85, 121

X

Xenograft tumor, 125

Printed in the United States
By Bookmasters